MULTIPLE SCLEROSIS

MULTIPLE SCLEROSIS

A Personal View

By

CYNTHIA BIRRER, M.A., B.Ed.

Director of Education
Pathways Institute of Thanatology

With a Foreword by

Lawrence D. Dickey, M.D.

Director
Continuing Medical Education Society
for Clinical Ecology

Illustrated by

William Birrer, M.Arch. (Penn)

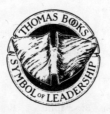

CHARLES C THOMAS • PUBLISHER
Springfield • Illinois • U.S.A.

Published and Distributed Throughout the World by
CHARLES C THOMAS • PUBLISHER
Bannerstone House
301-327 East Lawrence Avenue, Springfield, Illinois, U.S.A.

© *1979, by* CHARLES C THOMAS • PUBLISHER
ISBN 0-398-03864-3 (cloth)
ISBN 0-398-03886-4 (paper)
Library of Congress Catalog Card Number: 78-11340

With THOMAS BOOKS *careful attention is given to all details of
manufacturing and design. It is the Publisher's desire to present books that
are satisfactory as to their physical qualities and artistic possibilities and
appropriate for their particular use.* THOMAS BOOKS *will be true to those
laws of quality that assure a good name and good will.*

Printed in the United States of America
V-OO-2

Library of Congress Cataloging in Publication Data
Birrer, Cynthia.
    Multiple sclerosis, a personal view.

    Bibliography: p. 261
    Includes index.
    1. Multiple sclerosis--Biography. 2. Birrer,
Cynthia. 3. Multiple sclerosis. I. Title.
RC377.B57   362.1'9'6834   78-11340
ISBN 0-398-03864-3
ISBN 0-398-03886-4 pbk.

to my mother and father
who gave me tomorrow
yesterday

FOREWORD

CYNTHIA BIRRER in her MULTIPLE SCLEROSIS: A PERSONAL VIEW, exemplifies the concept of Clinical Ecology in operation. Clinical Ecology is a medical orientation which looks upon disease as an individual's specific reaction to environmental insults in terms of adaptation. Since individual susceptibility is a major component in this reaction, successful stabilization or reversal of this reaction depends upon the patient learning its nature and becoming able to identify the environmental excitants. Only in this way can they become the master of their destiny. It is not so much the physician as the patient's understanding and attitude that can modify the individual susceptibility factor.

Cynthia's self-determination, search for knowledge and recognition of ecologic factors in her case of multiple sclerosis helped to make it possible for her to cope with her problem. This she accomplished long before becoming aware of the concept of clinical ecology.

Clinical ecologists are approaching a wide range of physical and mental disorders of obscure origin and unfavorable prognosis using this concept. The concept is not new, but currently, because of the drug orientation of medical practice, it is not widely appreciated. The clinical ecology orientation for successful application is dependent upon the individual's willingness to alter his way of living, eating and even thinking in order to cope with environmental reaction.

This account of Cynthia's experience in coping with multiple sclerosis can be an inspiration to others suffering from disorders of obscure origin with an unfavorable prognosis.

Lawrence D. Dickey, M.D.
Fort Collins, Colorado

vii

Illness is a covenant which has its rule, its austerity, its silences and its inspirations.

Albert Camus

INTRODUCTION

10th December, 1975.

I GLANCED at my watch. 1:50 PM. Then I looked back across the desk at the solemn white-clad figure. Multiple sclerosis. Yes, that's what he had said. There was a sinking feeling deep down in the pit of my stomach. Because I knew — at least in so far as medical science is concerned — that, as yet, there is no cure for the disease. Did I really have an incurable disease? The doctor's voice came out of the gloom.

"In my opinion you do have multiple sclerosis. But I may be wrong. You must get confirmation."

18th December, 1975.

Once again I had told my long story, hesitantly. Again I had been examined, thoroughly, from head to toe. I waited, expecting the worst but hoping for a little better. But this doctor understood more clearly than I did then that I had a much better chance of achieving a realistic acceptance of my condition if he told me the truth. Kindly, but with no punches pulled.

"There is no possible alternative to the diagnosis of multiple sclerosis."

But still I hoped he might be mistaken. Although I could not see very well at the time nor could I personally visit the library, I read as much as possible about multiple sclerosis. Certainly it was considered by the medical profession to be incurable, but not immediately terminal.

Of course it meant that my very active life would have to be curtailed. As the disease progressed, bringing with it increased limitations of movement, I was persuaded that I would have to make adjustments, some of them quite radical. For a long time I had been experiencing difficulties with my speech and vision and hearing. I knew that life would not be easy and I did not, for one single moment, pretend otherwise. The time for playing games was over.

24th December, 1975.

I waited for the verdict of the third doctor.

"Mrs. Birrer, I agree with my two colleagues. I think their diagnosis is correct. In fact, it is the diagnosis I made on 18th November, which you were not told about."

Although I had prepared myself to hear these words of final confirmation, I felt devastated. Perhaps for the first time in my life I experienced real despair.

At home, I shut myself in my cosy, book-lined study. How could I cope with the pain of the knowledge that the plans I had made for myself over many years would have to be changed? How could I adapt so that my life would continue to be full and productive within the limitations of my disease? How could I deal with the pain that I knew my family and friends would feel as daily they watched my struggle with a disease that can bring with it many humiliations and indignities?

To be multiple sclerotic is to be sad. How we react to a diagnosis of multiple sclerosis is, in some ways, like the experience of bereavement, but instead of having lost a loved one through death, we have lost our good health and much besides through disease. It is not surprising, therefore, that all of us go through a long period of grief, perhaps as long as several years.

In that December, when I learned about my own loss, I experienced deep sadness, mingled with feelings of extreme anger and weak denial. I needed help then. I knew that I did and so did my family and friends. In the many days that have passed since then, I have met others, similarly afflicted, who need help too. Again and again I have pondered the nature of the help that we, being multiple sclerotic, need in order to become responsible for our own lives.

About 1800, the Danish philosopher Sorën Kierkegaard asked himself a similar question, and he found an answer, which is my own, and the inspiration for the pages that follow.

The secret of all helping, Kierkegaard says, lies in clearly understanding where the person who needs help really is: where she is to be found. This means that to help is, above all, to be able to put oneself in the place of the other, to make one's home in her existence, to get to know the world in which she lives: in short, to care.

To care for another person is to assist her growth. It is a process, a way of relating to someone that involves development, the desirable course to be taken by *this* human being in *this* situation. In caring as helping the other evolve, the person cared for is experienced as an extension of oneself, and at the same time as separate from oneself, worthy of respect in her own right. Thus the intrinsic direction of this person's development guides what is done, it determines how others are to respond and what is relevant to their response.

To help another person grow in this significant sense is at least to help her to care for something or someone apart from herself; that is, to help her find or create areas of her own in which she can care. Further, it is to enable her to come to care for herself, and through becoming responsive to her own inherent need to care, to accept a degree of responsibility for her life. Growing includes learning to the extent that one is able, where learning is the re-creation of one's person through the continual integration of new experiences and ideas. We develop by becoming more self-determining, and by choosing our values and ideals. We are more capable of making decisions and more willing to be responsible for them, and we can limit ourselves in order to discover and achieve what is truly important to us. We develop by becoming more honest with ourselves and more aware of the social and natural order of which each of us is an inseparable part.

. The problem is always how to care for this person here and now. To do this, we must come to understand her and her world as if we were inside it. We must be able to see, as it were, with her eyes what her world is like to her and how she sees herself. We must be with her in her world, "going" into it in order to sense from "inside" what life is like for her, what she is striving to be, and what she needs to develop.

Perhaps the only way to know this person is to go to the *things* of her world. *The relationship between a human being and her world is so intimate that they cannot be regarded apart.* If we try to do so, then human ceases to be human, and world to be world. Our world is not a conglomerate of objects, amenable only to the language of physical science or rational discourse. In fact, we seldom see actual objects, things as such; rather we grasp the significance they assume for us because our subjective condition is invested in them. My world is the materialisation of my essence. If you want to know me, listen to the language spoken by the things in my environment. Look at my home, my habitat, the livingscape within which I demonstrate and reveal myself.

Being multiple sclerotic means, in the first place, that I see the world differently. My surroundings have changed, invariably in some discouraging way. And this change is *real*, the absolutely literal expression of being multiple sclerotic. To understand the nature of this change you need to know, not how I feel, but how the world looks to me; how it, rather than me, has changed. For come what may, *I* do not change; despite the ravages of the disease I retain intact the identity that has been mine since birth and will continue to be mine after death.

But I do see that things are no longer the same and this different but true perception reflects the state of being multiple sclerotic. If you do not see things as I do it does not mean that your perceptions are more accurate, less distorted, than my own. All it means is that I am ill and you are not. But that you know already; more to the point is that you should discern my new reality so that we can share it.

To care and thus to help depends on your capacity to enter fully into the existence of this other who needs you. It is not to dominate or to dictate to her a way without some sense that it really can coalesce with her own existence.

With the loss of health comes another profound loss, one to which I was sure I could never be reconciled. During the monotony of the days and the tortuous hours of night I mourned deeply the loss of my independence, more precious to me than anything I possessed. Immobilised, near blind, I was dependent on others to meet every need. Had I been reminded then that we are all constantly dependent on things over which we have little or no control and that being multiple sclerotic only highlights this fact, I think I would have turned my face into my pillow and suffocated, literally as well as figuratively.

But almost imperceptibly the consistent caring of my family and friends helped me realise that what I was receiving in boundless measure did not have to be given; sick though I was I had no moral claim to anything beyond their attention to my basic needs, I could not legitimately demand more. I began to feel very close to what I depended upon, much as I depend on my books, the tools that have served me so well since that day long ago when I first learned to read. Now, instead of denying or, at most, grudgingly conceding my dependence on those around me, I feel joy in the ties that link us together. Only someone who helps others as a means of manipulating them experiences receiving help as imprisoning; she cannot take in because she fears being taken in.

And, too, I bitterly resented the peremptory loss of my career. Childless by choice, preferring to reach for a star in the academic firmament rather than shine in my own homely constellation, I did not anticipate much gold among the dross in the days to come. My life, it seemed, was over, a job half done. But again I found that being multiple sclerotic only amplifies the unfinished character of *all* living. Anyone who is growing and creating is always incomplete, in the making. As my present living began slowly to unfold, to expand and increase, I became acutely aware of the unfinished nature of living and of the importance of filling each minute, each hour, with real living.

The pain that comes with the loss of health through organic diseases takes many forms: physical, emotional, spiritual. But there is another kind of pain that I have to contend with. The searing, burning, lacerating pain of arachnoiditis. A raw and biting pain that cripples my body from lower spine to the very tip of my toes, a pain that is always there. A pain that is so intolerable during the dark nights that I hardly know how to endure it. A pain that is resistant to medical and surgical intervention. A pain that was caused by medical intervention: by a diagnostic procedure performed when I first consulted a neurologist. This pain is doctor-made, or iatrogenic.* Thus, I had another very serious lesson to learn: the dreamy wonders of science can sometimes turn into a ghastly blunder.

The pain, dysfunction, disability and anguish resulting from technical medical intervention now rival the morbidity due to traffic and industrial accidents and even war-related activities, and make the impact of medicine one of the most rapidly spreading epidemics of our time. Ivan Illich calls doctor-inflicted pain or infirmity *clinical iatrogenesis.*

There is, however, an equally noxious variety arising from the destruction by the health professions of the individual's potential to deal with his humanness — weakness, vulnerability, uniqueness — in a personal and autonomous way. It is called *cultural iatrogenesis,* and its effect is the paralysis of healthy responses to disease, suffering, pain and death.[43]

Not long ago, cultures fulfilled their hygienic function by transmitting the symbolic means for making pain tolerable, disease understandable, death meaningful. But the ideology of modern medicine runs counter to this function. It radically undermines the traditional folkways and prevents the creation of new patterns for self-care or healing in incurable disease.

Instead we meekly submit to a code formulated by the self-appointed custodians of our health. This is a technical program that denies each man's need to deal with pain, sickness and death. Modern medicine can tell us as much about the meaningful experience of suffering as chemical analysis tells us about the aesthetic value of pottery. Medicine is doing for people what their genetic and cultural heritage formerly equipped them to do for themselves. Suffering and dying, activities that culture once taught each of us, have been transformed into technical matters, devoid of personal meaning. And the body's own miraculous powers of healing that, until recently,

---

*(from the Greek, iatros = doctor; genesis = origin)

biological evolution guaranteed and jealously guarded, have been subverted.

But there is a new spirit abroad that found early expression in the spreading revolt against forced labour by women striving to give birth without violence. Striking the same note but in a different key is this montage of my experiences of the changes that suddenly confronted me when I became incurably ill. It is also a record of my struggle for adaptation; of the battle to take responsibility for living a healthy existence while yet being multiple sclerotic.

Obviously no one else can approach the disease in exactly the way I have done. There is always the difficulty of appropriateness to *this* novel situation; mimicking my experiences through a mechanical application of principles will not do. Every multiple sclerotic makes of the disease her personal reality, which is unique. But ahead of those embarking on the first stage of a journey that has a long course to wind, blooms many a rose among the thorns.

ACKNOWLEDGMENTS

> And one might therefore say of me that in this book I
> have only made up a bunch of other people's flowers,
> and that of my own I have only provided the string
> that ties them together.
>
> Michel de Montaigne

IN the jargon of the social sciences, that special kind of encounter that forms a context for the total redefinition of a person at different stages in the developmental cycle is called a *rite de passage*. This structured event allows the individual to confront, experience and express those powerful energies associated with matrices embedded deeply within the unconscious. In a sense, this book is such a rite of passage.

I, too, was assisted with my own long and lonely journey to transition following the diagnosis of multiple sclerosis by what others had written. If I have any extrasensory talent at all, it is in finding just the right book at exactly the right time. Thus I owe an immense debt to those whose spirit reached me through their words, playing a vital role in that magic transformation: Ivan Illich, J.H. van den Bergh, Oliver Sachs, Hans Selye, Milton Mayeroff, George Leonard, central among others.

Dr. Richard Mackarness was the first to crystallise my ecological ruminations, through his book *Not All in the Mind*. He introduced me to his American colleagues, among them Dr. Lawrence D. Dickey and Dr. William Rea, and I owe him more than he knows.

The Multiple Sclerosis Society of Rhodesia, in particular Mrs. Ray Rosenfeld and her husband, has shared its resources as well as understanding of multiple sclerosis.

The National Multiple Sclerosis Society of New York has also given unstintingly: almost by return post I received the MS

Home Care Program, vast quantities of literature and the MS READ-a-thon program.

Illustrations in this book, although original, are in some instances based in concept on those from *MS Home Care Course,* copyright © 1976 by the National Multiple Sclerosis Society and The American National Red Cross. These and paraphrased references to selected techniques are reproduced with permission.

I leave to last the members of the World Federation of Healers who at their conference in London in August, 1977, gave devotedly of themselves. To Gilbert Anderson first, and the others from the four corners of our globe who laid their hands in love upon me, from Bill and I: thank you. You were a pathway.

CONTENTS

MULTIPLE SCLEROSIS

SECTION I

Turning and turning in the widening gyre
The falcon cannot hear the falconer;
Things fall apart; the centre cannot hold
Mere anarchy is loosed upon the world,
The blood-dimmed tide is loosed, and everywhere
The ceremony of innocence is drowned;
The best lack all conviction, while the worst
Are full of passionate intensity.

Surely some revelation is at hand;
Surely the Second Coming is at hand
The Second Coming! Hardly are those words out
When a vast image out of Spiritus Mundi
Troubles my sight: somewhere in the sands of the desert
A shape with lion body and the head of a man,
A gaze blank and pitiless as the sun,
Is moving its slow thighs, while all about it
Reel shadows of the indignant desert birds
The darkness drops again; but now I know
That twenty centuries of stony sleep
Were vexed to nightmare by a rocking cradle,
And what rough beast, its hour come round at last,
Slouches towards Bethlehem to be born?

—William Butler Yeats, "The Second Coming."
Collected Poems. New York, Macmillan,
1924.

In the beginning . . .

AFTER a discordant night when sleep is light and fitfull, saturated by pervasive un-ease, I wake as dawn filters through the small window. I open my eyes, keep very still, hoping to lessen the rapid tautening of my right calf muscles. The spasm is violent and I gasp in pain. The second toe on the foot of the same leg is rigid. As by thongs the other four are drawn downward, stubby claws cruelly contorted. I freeze where I lie until my leg relaxes, eons later. I straighten the chill limb with consummate care, nauseous with relief at the passing of the contracture.

Something is the matter with me. Nevertheless, I get out of bed intending to start the day as usual. I take one step and stagger. On the second, I trip. With each I veer to the right. I steady myself against the door with the hand on that side. If I move forward my right leg will surely buckle at the knee.

I feel an eerie sense of dislocation as I catch the first brief glimpse of a world gone wrong. I go back to the bed I just left. The thermometer negates my action, unlike my queasy response to the inquiry about what I want to eat. I am sick. I give up my grapefruit and coffee as I give up everything the day is to bring, all my hopes and plans and duties. And to prove that I do so absolutely, I pull the blanket over my head.

Then, gradually, the irrevocable transmutation of being-ill takes place. I listen to the day unfold. From upstairs sounds of the quickening household reach the bedroom. The kitchen door bangs shut. Crockery en route to the table rattles; knives and forks clatter as they are coupled in their familiar settings. Petrus moves on soft feet through the north door onto the patio. Soon I hear the rhythmic swish, swish of his brush across its uneven surface. Our dog lumbers toward the dining room each step marked by claws clicking against ceramic floor tiles.

The telephone rings. Julia answers it and I listen.

I smell the day begin, too. Coffee percolating and toast charring. The acrid fumes of the first cigar. The sweetness of soap and shaving lotion and deodorant mingling in the nearby bathroom.

And I also hear that the day has begun out there in the street. Cars screech to a halt at the corner stop sign, then pull away. Motorcycles roar, one after another after another. School boys shout their tidings. Dogs bark furiously as a newspaper is delivered to each house. I have not heard the sounds of the morning like this for years.

How familiar and yet how strange it all is. How near and yet how far away things are. What I hear is the start of my daily existence. But there is a difference; I play no part in it. In a way, of course, I still belong completely to the happenings upstairs. I participate in all the noises I hear, all the odours I smell, but at the same time all of it passes me by, everything goes on at a great distance.

"Is Cynthia not feeling well?" My father's voice rises above the rustle of his newspaper. Even at this early moment, they have ceased to consider that I can hear them.

The bedroom door bursts open; Bill has come to say goodbye. He is remote. The distance I measured in the sounds I heard seems so much greater now that he is here, at my bedside, with his shaven face and immaculate suit and hurried gestures. Everything about him proclaims the normal healthy day, the day of work and leisure, of street and shop and office. The day outside this house, from which I am excluded, in which I have no place.

Multiple sclerosis

MULTIPLE sclerosis, or disseminated sclerosis, as it used to be called, is one of medicine's strangest mysteries, with an unknown cause, an unexplained geographic distribution, an unpredictable course, an undiscovered cure; while its treatment is, to say the least, highly controversial. Although the disease is nearly worldwide, it seems to be largely one of place, more prevalent in the Northern Hemisphere than in the Southern. As far as race is concerned, multiple sclerosis appears to be rare, if not absent, among blacks in Africa, but it occurs in similar frequency among black and white Americans. Thus it is associated with particular localities, rather than with any race living in these localities.

The symptoms start most often in adults from eighteen to forty years of age. In two-thirds of sufferers onset is between twenty and twenty-five; it is uncommon before fifteen or after forty-five. The age of onset is slightly younger in women than men, and they are more often victims of the disease. It is not hereditary, but it is familial.

Multiple sclerosis is a disease which affects the central nervous system — the brain and spinal cord. Through the transmission of impulses this controls such important functions as walking, talking, seeing and eating; tying a shoe lace and opening a door. The impulses travel along the nerve fibres in the central nervous system, then to the other parts of the body. Normally the nerve fibres are coated by a material called *myelin* which can be compared to the insulation around a telephone wire. Composed of fatty material and proteins, myelin permits nerve fibres to conduct impulses at rates up to 100 times faster than those not covered with it.

Not only is myelination incomplete at birth, but the processes of both brain growth and myelination proceed at

7

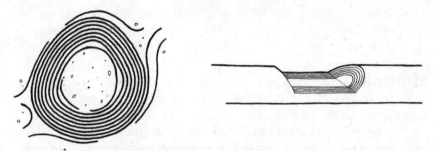

Figure 1 *(left)*. Greatly enlarged diagrammatic section through a nerve showing myelin layers wrapped around the nerve.
Figure 2 *(right)*. Greatly enlarged diagram showing myelin layers revealed by cutaway section.

different rates for different brain centres. The first areas of the cortex to become myelinated in the young infant are the motor control areas. Here the initial linkages are between the visual and motor areas, so that a baby under six months can both converge his eyes on an object and make limited movements towards it. At six months the sensory areas of the brain are more developed than at birth, but the sensory association areas remain undeveloped until the third year. Myelination of the nervous system is not complete until the early teens. We still do not know what factors promote optimum growth or, conversely, retard it.

One of the curious features of multiple sclerosis is that although we all have these sheaths around our peripheral nerves — in our arms and legs — the damage inevitably occurs only in our brains and spinal cords. The reason for this is not known; it is all part of the problem that has to be solved. But it is known that in multiple sclerosis changes around veins in certain areas of the central nervous system affect the myelin sheath. In effect, this is dissolved by some causative agent, so that the insulation is damaged; later the affected area is replaced by scar (sclerotic) tissue, from which the disease gets its name.

Early in the disease only the sheath is involved (primary demyelination), and the nerve fibres which it surrounds are not destroyed until later (secondary demyelination). If only the protective covering is diseased, the function of the fibres is impaired, but some impulses can still be transmitted, although not with full strength. Function is restored when the sheath's condition improves.

Once the nerve fibres themselves are replaced by scar tissue, called plaques, nerve impulses can no longer be carried. When a severe scar is formed it is difficult to see how the damage could be reversed, or what could do so. Consequently, with intense or prolonged impairment, function may be permanently lost in those parts of the body regulated by the damaged nerve fibres.

There are, nevertheless, other possibilities: for one thing, if the damage occurs in one particular nerve, say in one fibre of the optic nerve, it is possible that other nerve fibres can ultimately take its place. This may explain the waxings and wanings, the relapses and remissions, that are characteristic of multiple sclerosis: the remission marking the point at which other auxiliary nerve fibres take over the job that the damaged one had been doing. This alone presents two avenues of hope: to find a way to interfere with the scarring process, or to try to stimulate the formation of new myelin. This book is concerned primarily with the first possibility.

The reason why the disease is termed multiple is that almost any portion of the central nervous system may be involved. The spinal cord is perhaps the most frequently affected; this can cause periods of partial to complete paralysis of the legs and, at times, of the trunk and arms. With or without this weakness or paralysis, there may be lack of coordination, staggering and tremor, or poor coordination plus tremor of the extremities, and sometimes of the body and head.

Numbness, tingling and various sensory changes often occur. Eye symptoms are common, with involuntary movement of the eyeball, periods of double or blurred vision, even temporary to permanent blindness in one or both eyes. In advanced cases slurred speech and sometimes difficulty with bladder and bowel control are not unusual.

Quite often sufferers are euphoric. They seem unusally cheerful in spite of their incapacitating symptoms, or they continue to be hopeful and optimistic despite progressive impairment. On the other hand, many become severely depressed. In a few, there is loss of memory for recent events and deterioration in conceptual thinking.

Characteristically, the disease differs markedly from person to person, showing so much variation that it is difficult to forecast its course. Typically though, symptoms come and go in the beginning, occasionally disappearing completely. As the disease goes on, however, recovery may be less and less complete, with persistence and progression of symptoms. In a minority, less than 10 percent, multiple sclerosis has a relentless course without periods of remission; in others, the symptoms occur suddenly and persist with neither improvement nor progression; most often, relapses are mild and infrequent, separated by periods of five to fifteen years, permitting an active and full life. Dr. Reginald Kelly* recalls:

> I have met a woman who started with double vision at the age of twenty-two, who had ten incapacitating episodes following in rapid succession over the course of the next six weeks, and who was dead by the end of eight weeks. At the other end of the spectrum I remember another lady who had her first episode of double vision at the age of twenty-three on the first night of her honeymoon after eating for the first time in her life a lobster supper. She told me the next morning when she started to see double that she looked dispassionately at the two new experiences to which she had been subjected in the previous twelve hours and decided she could more easily reject the lobster for future enjoyment. She never ate lobster again.
>
> The second episode, from which also she recovered completely, was at the age of sixty-five. The third, from which again she recovered, was a paralysis following an abdominal operation at the age of seventy-one and she left the hospital with no neurological disability, to die at seventy-three from cancer.
>
> That is the other end of the spectrum and anything in

---

*Chairman of the Research Advisory Council of the Multiple Sclerosis Society, Great Britain; Physician-in-Charge, Department of Neurology, St. Thomas' Hospital; Physician of the National Hospitals for Nervous Diseases, London.

between can occur. It is interesting though, that the most common diagnosis on admission to the Royal Hospital and Home for Incurables in Putney, England, is multiple sclerosis. At that hospital all ages are accepted but the most common time interval between retreat to a wheelchair and admission to the hospital is three years. Yet the average of admission among patients with multiple sclerosis, when I last calculated it, was fifty-nine.

When looking at a young person in the first episode, one should therefore not look back to the girl of twenty-two who died in eight weeks. That is most exceptional. Rather think about what happens to the majority, in particular the lobster lady. Budget for a productive future, not for a fatalistic acceptance of no future at all.

I saw a young lady the other day who had been told by the chairman of the local Multiple Sclerosis Society that she must look at her future realistically and accept that she would never get out of a wheelchair, that she would never drive again and that she must give up all ideas of ever having a baby. Not only was the advice catastrophic, but it demonstrates the profound ignorance of the natural history of this disease.

Of course, there are those who have to cope with the grim realities of their own future as ordained by their personal experience of the disease when it shows them that they are among the unlucky few. But it is very difficult to judge when even they have reached the point of no return. I have known several who after ten years of a wheelchair existence have yet improved sufficiently to be able to travel on public transport once more. Let me hasten to add that this is not because of any treatment that I have been able to give. It is just that the disease behaves in this curious fashion.[44]

Clearly, then, multiple sclerosis is a disease which frequently runs an exceptionally benign course. One noted investigator reports that sixty-nine percent of men sufferers lived more than twenty-five, and 50 percent more than thirty-five, years after the onset, while death from the disease seemed to occur somewhat earlier in women than in men; for men the peak age of death was between sixty-five and eighty-four years.

In many of the cases that prove benign, the first lesion is

retrobulbar neuritis (inflammation of the nerves behind the eye), followed by a prolonged period of remission before other neurological symptoms develop; alternatively, an onset with sensory as distinct from motor symptoms seems to carry a good prognosis. But even those who suffer more frequent relapses and remissions, if their activity is relatively unrestricted within five to ten years after the first limb symptoms, the prognosis seems reasonably good. No rule is absolute, for one of the characteristics of this disease is its caprice. The important point is that whereas it was often said that multiple sclerosis was generally fatal within five to twenty-five years of its onset, in fact the course of the illness is more often remarkably benign.

The structural alterations that take place in the brain and spinal cord have been familiar to physicians for over a century. The written record of multiple sclerosis begins in 1822, when a young English nobleman, Sir Augustus D'Este, noted in his diary unmistakable evidence that he was a victim of some mysterious disease. When he died at the age of fifty-four, D'Este had spent at least twenty-six years of his life fighting this unseen enemy. In 1838, while D'Este was travelling all over Europe in a vain search for a cure, Sir Robert Carswell, a British medical illustrator, included in his *Pathological Anatomy* a watercolour of a strange-looking spinal cord he had seen during an autopsy. On the otherwise seemingly healthy cord were scattered spots of hardened and discoloured tissue. Carswell described the condition as "a peculiar diseased state of the spinal cord accompanied by atrophy of the discoloured portions."[20]

Almost at the same time a French physician, Jean Cruveilhier, observed similar spots on the spinal cord at the autopsy of a woman who had been hospitalized for many years. He called the spots "islands of sclerosis," from the Greek for "hardening," and speculated that they might have actually caused the disease. Thirty more years were to pass before multiple sclerosis was properly identified.

It was Jean Martin Charcot, one of France's most famous medical investigators, who in 1868 gave the world a detailed description of the disease. Working at the Salpêtrière hospital in Paris, Charcot found that many of his patients were suffering from varying degrees of tremor and paralysis. Some of these patients suffered from the shaking palsy, which had been first described by James Parkinson in England in 1817. Charcot realised, however, that another distinct disease was present, evidenced by tremor and varying degrees of spastic paralysis, or stiff and jerky body and limb movements. At autopsy victims of this disease showed plaques, or hardened flat patches, scattered throughout the central nervous system. He called the disease *Sclérose en plaques.*

Charcot found that patients frequently experienced alternating exacerbation and remission of symptoms, that the severity of the symptoms varied greatly from patient to patient and that often the illness appeared to remain stationary for many years. In its advanced stages he found that the disease was characterised by paralysis and by three additional symptoms now known as Charcot's triad. One of these is *intention tremor:* the limbs, particularly the arm and hand, shake violently whenever the person tries to control his movements. The second symptom is slow and *scanning speech,* where there is a pause after each syllable. The third is ocular abnormalities, particularly *nystagmus,* an involuntary flicking of the eye back and forth, up and down or around and around.

From the time of Charcot, many important contributions to the literature of multiple sclerosis rapidly increased. But although it has been known as a pathologic entity for over 150 years and as a clinical disease for more than 100; has been subjected to intensive, exhaustive and multifaceted investigation; today most of its mysteries remain unsolved.

. . . the next day . . .

THE onset of multiple sclerosis signals a halt. Life, as one has known it, is at an end. Another world has taken its place, a base world, simpler and starker than the old one. It is impossible to give this world a substance of its own, or to conceive what its sorrows and sufferings, or joys, might be.

When I am able to venture into the city, the buildings are immense. Imperturbable, solid, they contrast strongly with the uncertainty I feel, the frailty of my wasting body, my hesitant steps. Looking skyward I see that they lean toward each other so that the clear blue strip between the sombre concrete columns is much narrower than the unyielding slabs on which I carefully position my unfeeling feet.

The streets are alarmingly wide. I am quite certain that I cannot get across this one. My legs, which are unsure in familiar surroundings, would betray me altogether if I attempt to do so.

The multitudes scurrying along the pavements are more crowded and dense than that narrow space actually allows. Yet when a figure brushes against me, the fleeting sense of claustrophobia gives way immediately to the impression of a vast space between us. I am wholly isolated and at the same time grow more and more afraid. Again and again fear forces me to return, task undone, until eventually it keeps me from going out at all.

From the safe womb of my study, the street, the crooked alleys of the shopping mall, the shallow stairs rising endlessly in the dim light of the cinema present a less daunting aspect. But even in seclusion, just contemplating the breathless bustle of the world outside is sufficient to induce a heavy sense of dread. Less and less can I make the effort to forsake the fa-

14

miliar. Now it is impossible to escape my nightmare impressions of the smallest suburban shopping centre, the cosiest restaurant, the friendliest gathering. Each notation of an event in my diary represents a Pandora's box of undefined and inexplicable terrors. This is the way I see things and they are ominous. I am so fearful of them that they make me a recluse, confined within the boundaries created by the white garden wall.

Today, my world is shrunken to the size of my bedroom, or rather my bed. Even going to the bathroom is an unfriendly, slightly surreal excursion. From the toilet, on which I find myself seated very often, the patterned wall tiles which I noticed vaguely, if I ever saw them at all, have to be meticulously analysed in small and large figures. I am compelled to scrutinise the pattern, symmetric here, asymmetric there, and to detect in it caricatures of people and animals and things. I am obsessed by the upturned snouts of the profusion of pigs. It is like taking a huge Rorschach test. Weird interpretations insinuate themselves, particularly when I feel helpless and alone. And I want to cry when I find a curve or a line that stubbornly resists the design that demanded so much effort.

My clothes, hanging from hooks at the back of the bedroom door, are another reminder that the limits of my existence are crushingly circumscribed. The black slacks and the ribbed body shirt belong to the outside world. I see myself ascending the stairs beyond my bedroom, going to work, in the library, receiving guests. Certainly I am that woman, yet at the same time I have ceased to be her. The clothes are very near, but they belong to a time that is gone. I feel deep attachment, even a longing for those clothes. They speak of my other being, of a reality that must have had its value. Yet if the meaning of a life depends on working eight hours each day, five days a week in a total institution, it could not mean too much. I am relieved then when loving hands change my bedroom into a proper sickroom and my clothes are put away in the wardrobe. For no matter how gentle the reminder is, I do not like to be reminded at all: there is nothing that I can do to regain that other existence.

My horizon is the edge of my bed. But even this intimate repository is no longer wholly my domain. When I knew the interminable rhythm of work and sleep, of being up-and-about and of being in-bed, my bed was an attribute of the night. At day's end the world narrowed to our lounge. The drawn curtains enclosed my being by myself or our being together. When I got into bed the world narrowed to my bed. Aired by breezes which daily blew through the open windows, it received me with consistent hospitality. I made it my own, stretching, seeking comfort for my arms and legs, and solace for my head upon the pillow. Tomorrow was the span I created between all things and myself. The world was quiet. Sleep arrived. Sleep was the contraction of my existence; I lost myself within myself. But everything would return to me tomorrow. Sleep was the promise of the future.

Now apart from the exact spot where I lie my bed is cold and rejecting. The pillow welcomes me just where my head touches it. Each move is an achievement, a minor conquest. Sleep is elusive because what is to come tomorrow is only my bed and that is not a promise; it is a permanent confinement. Now, too, sleep is not being-contracted. That is impossible because the movement outward into the world, the being-expansive, is absent. The stale smell of sheets and pillow and pyjamas reminds me of a reductive existence which knows no change.

My bed is my abode for hours each day and for days at a stretch. My blankets, articles of utility which once lacked character and colour, are jungles of matted pink skeins through which my eye roves ceaselessly. The sheets are vast flowery plains with valleys and slopes and summits, a spring pasture to the paralysed traveller that I am. My bed is the place that eventually I may never leave, or may exchange occasionally for a wheelchair. It is the marital bed, the place of procreation; how soon will it be a deathbed?

My visitors affect my experience of my sickbed. For me it is never an accepted fact; it is always an emergency. But for them this is obviously not the case. Sometimes they come into my room and speak of the things that happen outside as if they are describing a foreign land that I may never see again. They talk about the life that a short time ago was mine in a way that implies that I have ceased to be a part of it. I am merely a patient. Everywhere my place is taken by others.

It is not only words that openly announce my demise. It has also to do with intonation, of the way my visitor sits next to my bed and his manner of leaving. These intangible qualities of each visit enlarge the void between the worlds of health and disease that I know too well, and would love to see diminish with the arrival of someone who is not multiple sclerotic.

Visitors are an implicit invitation to participate in that other world, at least by way of conversation, but this is often what mine deny me. Some enter my room in a tearing hurry, mention a dozen things in a few moments and then disappear. When, alone, I try to recapture their hasty words and mull them over, I am confused, perplexed, dejected. They do not intend to wound me, but actually I am hit where it hurts the most. The harsh reality that brings them to my bed in the first place, and my detention in a room outside of which life goes on easily and sensibly, are heavily underscored. I am a member of a lesser caste.

Another visitor remains standing beside my bed so that the freedom of easy dialogue is lost. Inevitably much of what he says is addressed to the wall. I am equally disadvantaged when my visitor moves his chair close to my bed. He leans over me, encroaching upon the decent measure between two people talking. My location is fixed so I cannot move backward, or find another position to protect the space I consider my own. Sometimes I am unable to move myself at all.

Then there are those who sit on my bed or sprawl all over it, so that every word uttered seems like an earthquake. "How is everything?" they ask. They barely expect a reply. If I do try to explain how things are, how those things are which hurt and tear at me, my words hardly reach them.

I lack the courage to voice these feelings because I may upset my visitors and deter them from another visit. After all, I depend upon people coming to me. I cannot return the compliment; our status is no longer equal. I always feel indebted to those who do come, especially as they rarely appear empty-handed. This reduces my freedom in our contact even further. It is exhausting to be grateful for every piece of fruit, for the flowers for which there is hardly any room left, and for the book that only increases the heap of literature with which my failing sight can no longer cope. Fatigued beyond recrudescence, I ask my doctor to set a limit on the time they can stay with me.

I thought, in the beginning, that my departure would create problems. Now these problems are no longer apparent. No one seems to worry about them, least of all my old colleagues. Things are going pretty well without me; I am not needed anymore. So little do people miss me that now my absence is not even noticed. They only remember when the calendar says that it is time to pay Cynthia another visit.

And so the noises from the street; the noises in the house; the new way in which the light filters through the windows in the morning and gives way to artificial light in the evening; the new appearance of my room with the too large bouquet of flowers and the too expensive basket of assorted goodies; the way my visitors come and speak and act — all these things teach me that life outside my small existence has become distinctly exotic.

. . . the day after . . .

UNDER other circumstances, before I became multiple sclerotic, I lived in the future, and in the past only in so far as it affected my future. Apart from a few special moments, I never really lived now: of present living I knew little, I gave it no thought. But incurable disease denies me escape: multiple sclerosis focuses and crystalises the eternal present.

All of existence is immediate now. This is quite a discovery for someone pledged to the future. Before I was multiple sclerotic, I was not conscious of my body; it performed its tasks like an expertly programmed computer. I passed on to it the duties it had to do and they told me that I have a body. The steering wheel of my car revealed my hands to me; the gear lever the strength of my arms; the pedals the smooth response of my feet; grassy slopes the fragility of my legs. Paper and pen showed me the dexterity of my right hand and the awkwardness of my left. Music confirmed my hearing and literature and art my vision. And when I looked at my body I recognised everywhere the marks and signs of its duties: bruises, scars, freckles.

Being multiple sclerotic I find that my body is something more than an overcoat, the purely material encasement of what I really am. In this state I cannot avoid the reality that I am my body. I am not consoled by the remark that my illness has only to do with my physical shell; I know, as you cannot, that my whole existence is stricken by a calamity.

Long ago a mother's hand bathed and swaddled my body, and through her loving gestures I learned to dwell in it. As she held me with her hands, eyes, voice, smile, I learned too how to contain myself, how to attend to the people and things in my infant world. Now, sitting beside my sickbed she touches my arm; she does not touch a sheath which, somehow, contains her child. The soothing contact of hand on arm is the contact of

19

two human beings, without any barrier, direct, an immediate participating in one another.

The gentle hand which caressed my body from birth and the affectionate touches, gave me the wonderful sense that my body is good. I respected it and I expected that others would too. But for the doctor my body belongs to a different world, one of physical dimensions. My body is a thing which I possess, a thing he can analyse and explain.

Thus, before we understood the meaning of my strange symptoms, a procedure called myelography was performed on my body. I did not then appreciate the risks that were involved. "There is no such thing as a safe myelogram," a Swedish professor told me later.

The neurologist did it to find an explanation for my deteriorating sight and stumbling gait. Iophendylate was introduced into my spinal canal because it is easy to visualise on an X-ray plate. This is a chemical of some value. It is radiopaque and oily, providing in rare instances critical information. Before the slipped disc was recognised in 1934 as a cause of low back pain and sciatica there was little need for myelography except to diagnose cord tumours. Few myelograms were done and the possible hazards of the dye were accepted as a legitimate risk in exchange for an accurate diagnosis in these rare cases. But many neurosurgeons admit that today the dye is often used when it is not clearly indicated, and is harmful. After all, it is they who dig about in the soggy mess that is the cauda equina of some unfortunate in whom five or ten cubic centimetres of iophendylate was optimistically injected a year or two previously. Not only is the original disease still there, but on top a chronic, adhesive, chemical inflammation of the caudal roots is engrafted.

Lying on my back I am in contact with my bed along the length of my body. At its base my spine flares. Both buttocks burn. The right lower limb is fiery, the left one less so. The soles of my feet are scorched. Even if my legs were strong enough, I could not move about on that lacerated flesh. Each flare-up reminds me of the contempt for my nervous system bred in the mind of that neurologist by the riotous expansion of medical technology. I may never forget as I lie here that among the men who should have ultimate regard for the human body are those who cannot be trusted.

My brain and spinal cord were given to me originally in full complement. Not only cannot one single damaged nerve cell be replaced, but even healing, beneficient elsewhere, is noxious here. Healing by scar to close a gap in bone or skin or muscle is a saving property. But in the nervous system, scar from injury or inflammation can only interfere with blood supply and function of the normal territory adjacent. The simple truth is that there is no regeneration of the tissues of the central nervous system.

Now that I am sick and in great pain my body is frequently foreign to me. It has become unfaithful. Knife and fork emphasize effete hands. The legs that bore me are recalcitrant. My sight is capricious, my hearing sporadic. The trusted ally has become a protagonist, an agonising foe. The caressing hands which gave my body to me and shaped my feelings towards it, and which still desperately try to overcome its infidelity, are powerless. Arachnoid pain, my constant companion, has excised their effect.

Opposite my bed on the wall above the heater is a woodcut of the crucifixion. It was executed by my great-grandfather using a special technique he perfected. I always felt ambivalent about it, vaguely embarrassed by the topic which had no firm foothold in my life. During the days when I could move very little, my room froze. The heater burned constantly, darkening the wood, or so I thought. It seemed that the lights of Jerusalem far beneath the horizontal beam of the cross, dimmed. As my own pain rose to new levels the thin figure, pitifully stretched and wrenched, began to radiate anguish and torment beyond description. I cannot now imagine a more poignant expression of human suffering.

In consequence, I am acutely aware of bodily existence. Often it makes itself felt in a general malaise, in un-ease or dis-ease. My body that was the unacknowledged condition of my being has become the pivot of my attention. My present, which served the future and was an effect of the past, is consumed by my awareness of myself. But I do not find the significance of my body on the outside; now it clamours within. This body is not an instrument, a condition, but an object, a prey to disease. It is a thing that is probed and palpated by the doctor. Multiple sclerotic, I live with a defunct body in a disjointed present.

I am fundamentally denied. Present living is felt not to be enough because I cannot use my own special gifts. Being multiple sclerotic I am kept from the lecture room, as from everything else. I no longer experience myself as competent. I feel outside life, as if it were passing me by, because I have no vital engagement in it.

The present stretches as a desert where nothing grows and nothing is of value. I cannot animate anything or be animated by anything. Reflecting on the past and future aggravates the emptiness and futility of the present. Because I am unable to make significant contact with my environment, there is a contraction of self. Life is devoid of purpose; there is nothing I wish to serve, nothing to explore that might make me receptive to more creative ways of living. Life lacks promise: no matter what I do, no matter what happens, the deadly stasis continues. My distinctive powers are negated and I am unfree.

Chronic pain

Pain loses its referential character if it is dulled and generates a meaningless, questionless residual horror.

Ivan Illich[43]

CHRONIC pain is a continuing condition rather than a clearly delineated interlude; it often has no forseeable end and a barely remembered beginning. It crowds consciousness and its effects are all-embracing: emotional pain, most typically a mixture of anxiety and depression; social pain, accompanying the gradual loss of responsibilities for children not yet independent, or for a partner who has provided lifelong support; spiritual pain, the feeling of meaninglessness and the desperate search, the struggle to make "a raid on the inarticulate"; and physical pain, introducing unscalable barriers into thought and action.

Chronic pain in multiple sclerosis, whether intrinsic to a particular case, or doctor-inflicted, is diffuse like a wave, with a predilection for the lower back and the extremities beyond. It is incoercible pain, a violent explosion at a definite point in time, tearing, shooting, rasping, gnawing, throbbing, burning. This pain is an inescapable fact of consciousness and its intensity seems to harmonise with the whole of my life now, fluctuating but never absent.

Even though my skin is anaesthetic, light contact, a slight variation in temperature, the merest pressure, provoke an excruciating exacerbation of it. The acuteness of my perception of my pain has nothing to do with the quantity of this aggravation; no matter what, the pain immediately reaches its summit, persisting long after the disturbance has ceased. Irrespective of the nature of these intrusions, they are all integrated into the experience of absolute pain: a banging door, an acrid smell, a doleful symphony, bright lights, emotional upsets. Incidents haphazardly jumbled into pain that does not diminish, pain unperturbed by any treatment.

My pain belongs in a unique way to me, so that I am utterly alone with it. I cannot share it. I have no doubts about the reality of my unceasing experience of pain, but I cannot really tell you about it. You can observe the outward signs of my pain but my inner experience of pain will always be invisible to you. It is this awareness of extreme loneliness in the midst of pain as one of the truest facts of human existence that sets the experience of chronic pain apart from any other. I realise with a sense of shock that all inner experiences, most more subtle than chronic pain, pervading our lives, are invisible, inaccessible. Since these are the most real part of us, *every* other experience, regardless of level of being, is invisible.

As I endure my pain, I am also aware that a question is being asked that is as much a part of chronic pain as my loneliness. Pain tells me about something not answered, something that time and again starts to scream: What is wrong? How much longer? Why must I suffer? Why, in God's name, does this kind of hell exist? What have I done to invite this evil? But his training has made the doctor adept at side-stepping pain's clamorous questions; he refuses to entertain them, and so I have to dig deep to uncover a possible symptom of health in the capacity to suffer. His avid concern with those aspects of pain that can be managed, more or less, by drugs or surgery make incomprehensible or shocking any ideas I might have that skill in the art of suffering could possibly be the most effective way of dealing with my pain.

Allopathic medicine is concerned with pain as a systemic reaction that can be verified, measured and regulated. Doctor and sufferer alike are interested only in medical methods of control, not an approach that might help the person in pain accept responsibility for her experience. Instead, pain has created a vociferous demand for more pain killers, hospitals and medical services to promote artificially induced insensibility and, ineluctably, clinical iatrogenesis.

Moreover, the medical profession has become the sole arbiter of which pains are authentic, which have a physical and which a mental base, which are imagined and which are simulated. Our society recognises and endorses this professional judgment, and the person in pain is left with less and less subjective and intersubjective context to give meaning to the experience that often overwhelms her. With indecent haste and incredible success, cultural iatrogenesis is stripping us of the classical, vital constituents of our humanness.

The doctor thinks and works as if my nervous system is the seat of reflexes and of purely intellectual processes, nothing else. He has forgotten, if he ever knew, that whatever the causes or the consequences of my pain, whether these are manifest in the end in biochemical, physiologic, psychologic or social terms, *first* they must be initiated in my central nervous system. Surely this imposes on him the strictest necessity to protect and preserve my nervous system — to be aware, at least, that where lurks the merest hint of a diagnosis of multiple sclerosis, that masked intruder, certain investigatory procedures are to be strictly avoided?

Morality in medicine

THE practice of medicine — what does it mean? Broadly, the diagnosis by examination, and the treatment of a condition of ill health. Whether general practitioner or specialist, the doctor acts as a clinician whenever he treats a patient. His treatment rests on his clinical judgment, which is largely a matter of what he knows of, rather than about, patients; what he knows of the things that can be learned only in the course of caring for the sick.

In all diseases, the outcome in a given situation depends at any specific time upon the interactions among the sick individual (her genetic predisposition and acquired state of health), the medical environment (investigatory procedures, drugs, etc.) and the quality of the mode of transmission (the doctor). This means that the nature, frequency and severity of the complications of modern medical practices are entirely the result of the relationships between the patient, the doctor and his interventions.

Clearly, then, the doctor performs an experiment every time he treats a patient. During a single week of active practice a busy clinician conducts more experiments than most medical researchers do in one year. This argument is consistent with the definition offered by Claude Bernard, a founder of experimental discipline in medicine. Said Bernard, "We give the name experimenter to the man who applies methods of investigation, whether simple or complex, so as to make natural phenomena vary, or so as to alter them with some purpose or other . . ."[6] Bernard was mainly interested in probing disease mechanisms, but his definition also covers the doctor's work in therapeutic management.

Prescribing drugs and investigatory procedures are the most common and perhaps pernicious forms of modern medical experimentation. One reason for this is that there is "no drug with a single action and there is no patient with a single type of response."[92] Under similar circumstances (dose, route of administration, technique, etc.) the reactions of different individuals will be different.

Although clinical and laboratory experiments are similar in some respects, there are important differences between them. The experimental material in a laboratory is an intact animal, a part of a person or of an animal, or an inanimate system. This is selected without regard to its desire or consent for participation and the experiment is initiated whenever the experimenter chooses. In clinical therapy, on the other hand, the material is an intact human being who herself initiates the experiment by seeking medical assistance. In volunteering as a subject for therapy she chooses the time and place, as well as the doctor who will serve as the investigator.

Recently, concern about the ethics of laboratory experiments has extended beyond the medical profession to philosophers, lawyers and other students of human morality. Conversely, the morality of experiments conducted in a clinical setting is rarely questioned. For one thing, these are seldom recognised as "experiments"; for another the procedures followed by the clinician are accepted by both the medical and lay public as well established and capable of replication without untoward variation.

But what "mode" of "therapy" is, in fact, truly "established"? We are expected to have confidence in our doctor's choices — but what choices can doctors themselves really be confident about? Many features of contemporary therapy are not replicable, lack validation and are by no means universally regarded as well established. In Norway and many other European countries, for example, the disadvantages of iophendylate are considered to be so significant that this medium is rarely used. The Swedish health authorities prohibit its use in the subarachnoid space.[36] In South Africa, on the other hand, a radiologist says, amid an assenting chorus, that he considers iophendylate to be a very safe substance which, presumably, would not harm a fly.[81] As a matter of fact, chemicals as inocuous as pest strips can and do result in severe reactions — that is, in chemically susceptible humans, especially ones with central nervous system or musculoskeletal symptoms, as well as in other assorted pests. "At a time of potent drugs and formidable surgery, the exact effects of many therapeutic procedures are dubious and shrouded in dissension — often documented either by the unquantified data of "experience" or by grandiose statistics whose mathematical formulations are so clinically naive that any significance is purely numerical rather than biologic."[25]

These extraordinary contradictions in clinical practice are generally ignored by the layman as well as the medical practitioner. The former, mesmerised by the magnificent equipment, expensive research and plethora of drugs, is convinced that the clinician *must* be making colossal advances. The medical profession, fully cognizant that the bulk of our problems are likely to elude "scientific" solution for many years to come, allows the doctor to justify what he does in terms of hunches, intuition or clinical experience. "His decisions are allowed a rationale that need not be overly rational, and reasons that need not be particularly reasonable. If the clinician seems knowledgeable and authoritative, and if his reputation and results seem good, he can be condoned the most flagrant imprecisions, vagueness and inconsistency in his conduct of therapy."[25]

The clinician calls the way he designs, executes and appraises his therapeutic experiments "clinical judgments." Surely no disease illustrates more clearly the hazards of hasty investigatory procedures and ill-conceived prescriptions, or is more liable to the mind-boggling fallibilities of clinical judgment, than multiple sclerosis. Few people suffer as much as multiple sclerotics while the doctor draws together a bewildering array of often wildly disparate symptoms under that enigmatic medical umbrella, his clinical judgment.

The traditional but utterly false doctrine that clinical judgments are too saturated by the complexities inherent in *any* human situation (lawyers and teachers are as likely to come up against them as doctors) to permit a high degree of accuracy grants them an unwarranted immunity from critical examination and assessment. It is also the lame plea doctors commonly make to normalise their errors — which, as far as multiple sclerosis is concerned, are often outrageous — thereby transforming them by sleight of hand from legitimate sources of liability into mere differences of opinion.

The doctor does not see professional mistakes in the same light as we do. He argues that normal, excusable mistakes occur through lack of information, the uncertainty of medical knowledge, the limitation of available techniques and the uniqueness of the case. The average doctor would not even call these mistakes: they are unavoidable events, suffered or risked rather than omitted or committed. They do not reflect competence, but luck. In consequence, no doctor will judge or criticise a mistake of this nature by a colleague because "there but for the grace of God go I." Laymen, understandably, are much less inclined to accept the idea of normal, excusable mistakes since they are the ones who have to live with their effects.

Deviant mistakes are distinguished from those which are normal and acceptable. Doctors do consider these to be due to a practitioner's negligence or ignorance, and that they reflect upon his lack of basic or reasonable competence, ethicality, conscientiousness and judgment. Such a mistake occurs because of the ubiquitous pressure in medicine to take some immediate action. A doctor's judgment is therefore evaluated in terms of what evidence was available at the time of his action, and not what is or could have been known after the fact.

In these circumstances, judgment becomes a synonym for "a matter of opinion"; there is no stable criterion for decision so that, within the general limits of known alternatives, every decision is equally correct at the time it is made. "Only the outcome allows talk of 'error': in the decision-making process itself at the time it occurs, there can be only different opinions, not mistaken choices."[30] Thus the glaring fact of the error is neutralised or normalised; an "error" which would cost any other professional his reputation and his livelihood miraculously becomes an "opinion."

By emphasizing the complexity of the problem as well as the ambiguity of the evidence, the "clinical judgment" of a doctor is able to make a deviant error honest, intelligible and, so, excusable. A mistaken decision taken at a specific point in time can be legitimately interpreted as a matter of opinion. Except in the most blatant cases, "judgment" removes any real reproach from the acknowledgment of a mistake, since differences in opinion do not call the doctor's competence into question.

Eliot Freidson, a noted medical sociologist, finds that it is almost a ritual, perhaps a way of diluting censure by oneself or others, for doctors to say that they learned something from their mistake and that the same mistake will not happen again. Nevertheless, the ambiguous nature of the data that is responsible for the honest error, in the first place, remains. Moreover, if a doctor can actually learn something from his mistake, perhaps he is now aware of something he should have known before, in which case his error is much less honest than he claims. Certainly, it is not something that could have "happened to anyone."

The whole idea of clinical judgment is suspect. Above all, it virtually prohibits the use of consistent rules, technical and ethical, to evaluate and control mistakes. Without these, any criterion on which to assess performance becomes so permissive that an intolerable range of variation creeps in. Only the grossest acts of incompetence and inattention, which all doctors would recognise and condemn, remain securely in the category of deviant mistakes. However, these are highly improbable in any sane doctor with an average medical training. Anything at all beyond this can be normalised, and responsibility for it evaded. Such acts may be mistakes or errors, deviations from standard practice (assuming that the standard practice itself is not deviant), but they do not justify sanctions.

This unlimited flexibility in the practice of medicine calls for an attitude of humility, even ignorance. Doctors are not particularly noted for either. Evidence regarding the long- and short-term effects of diagnostic and therapeutic interventions is inevitably ambiguous. This should serve to make doctors acutely aware that their own acts may have unforeseen consequences, and not as a loophole through which they slip with uncanny alacrity. Even though no doctor can know exactly what these effects will be, every doctor most certainly knows that an intervention need not realise its intended purpose.

Indeed, most errors in medical practice are not due to incompetent performance of prescribed treatment or to the violation of medical ethics or dereliction out of greed or laziness; these are the traditional charges to which doctors were vulnerable. The damage inflicted by the modern doctor occurs in the ordinary practise of well-trained men and women who accede to prevailing professional judgment and procedure even though they know (or could and should know) what damage they do.

The depersonalisation of diagnosis and therapy by the advent of a technology of awesome proportions has made malpractice a technical, not an ethical, problem. What was once considered an abuse of confidence and a moral fault is now rationalised as the unavoidable breakdown of equipment and operators. Today negligence is "random human error" or "system failure," callousness is "scientific detachment," and incompetence "a lack of information or specialised equipment."[43]

These dangers are magnified where doctors form their opinions and attitudes on social or religious, and *not* purely medical, grounds. Often the issue is ostensibly of a technical nature, and there are defined legal circumstances when it definitely is technical. More usually, however, it is primarily nonmedical and the attitudes of doctor and layman alike derive from some or other aspect of social morality in general. Medical expertise as such does not enter into the picture; and medical ethics, rooted in the Hippocratic Oath, are confined to the medical profession, which is a minority group regardless of its disproportionate power. Medical morality is not binding on laymen and often is not acceptable to them. Many, for instance, believe that the universal principle of truth-telling, particularly when it relates to what is going on in their own bodies, supersedes the more limited principle of patient interests, particularly when that is seriously prejudiced by the doctor's other nonmedical considerations, whether conscious or unconscious. Both the Soviet Union and South Africa provide examples of doctors who subvert the interests of their patients to that of the State, for example.

Despite the nonmedical nature of many problems which arise within the medical sphere of influence, law courts accept the testimony of doctors to the exclusion of the testimony of laymen. In Anglo-Saxon and Roman-Dutch law hearsay evidence is not admissible in court. This rule was established to keep the theologian and the inquisitor out of court. Over the years an exception was made to this maxim in favour of the so-called expert witness. In effect, the man with the secret knowledge has come back into the courtroom.

The obvious fact that the "expert" testimony of the doctor is generally based on the same broad social concerns as the attitudes of the layman is completely ignored. This makes it doubtful whether a doctor's evaluation of patient care, for instance (apart from its restricted technical details), is better informed than that of a layman; or whether how much a person must be told in order to be informed for her consent to some action taken on her body ought to be determined by what other doctors would have disclosed in similar circumstances. What, precisely, is inherently medical about deciding how much attention to basic human needs is required, or how much information a person would want to know? Whether or not an individual has received either adequate care or sufficient information is a question of *fact*, to be judged by the standards of a reasonable man, not those of a technocratic elite. To hold otherwise would permit the medical profession to determine its own responsibilities.

Moreover the testimony of a doctor in such cases is likely to be anything but expert. How can it be when it is based on moral positions common to both physician and layman? Nor is it likely that these will differ much in sophistication since the emphasis of a doctor's training is technologic skill and not sensitivity to points of social morality.

Since doctors have an undue influence on the resolution of fundamental sociomedical issues, it is important to understand the moral grounds on which their decisions rest. The thalidomide tragedy instigated fresh debates over the morality of abortions, infanticide and euthanasia more generally. These have taken place largely among doctors who firmly believe that they are discussing questions of medical morality. In so far as the debates concern a moral issue within a medical context, medical morality is involved. But it is not peculiarly medical norms and values that constitute the core of the disputations; it *is* medical norms and values, however, which are often at the heart of crucial differences between doctor and layman.

Earl Babbie found, in his study of science and morality in medicine, that when physicians discuss the morality of infanticide, they do not speak as medical men, their opinions are not drawn from specifically medical concerns. Rather they speak as religious men and irreligious men. In short, their opinions and those of the layman are informed by identical factors. "A very religious Catholic physician and a very religious Catholic plumber are both likely to oppose infanticide as immoral. The source of their opposition is to be found in their shared religious perspective, however, not in medicine or in plumbing."[3]

Morality in medicine, therefore, reflects predominantly social as opposed to medical concerns. In framing opinions on an ostensibly medical issue, doctors are influenced more by social than medical morality. Their perspectives are steeped in broad social and philosophical views, not professional training and experience. In other words, other things being equal, a good man will make a good doctor. Regardless of what he does or does not learn in medical school, he will know that with any procedure he undertakes or any drug he prescribes the chances of benefit must preponderantly outweigh the potential harm or injury — Hippocrates' first dictum, which the modern doctor seems to have lost sight of altogether. In an editorial in *Surgery, Gynecology and Obstetrics* pleading for respect for the tissues of the central nervous system where damage is irreversible, Dr. Eric Oldberg cautions: "When in doubt — don't risk it!"[66]

. . . yesterday . . .

> What has passed, has gone
> What is past, will come.
>
> Martin Heidegger

THE past is the storehouse of everything I have given form to, of immutably materialised possibilities; while the future comprises opportunities yet to be realised. My past is that part of my life wherein I overcame the essential transitoriness of human existence. Only under the urge and pressure of life's ephemeras does it make sense to use time. Actually, though, the only passing aspects of life are its potentialities. As soon as one is realised it becomes an actuality. Thus it remains an inviolable treasure, irrevocably stored, rather than irrevocably lost.

Since I found access barred to the state of being well, it has begun to beckon me with urgency and new promise. The world grows dearer and more vivid; it acquires an intimacy that is amazing. Daily trifles are more desirable than ever before. I have discovered another life of astonishing intensity. Once wholly occupied by the important matters of career, learning, esteem, I overlooked the little things. Now I have a fresh sense for these. I know the rhythm of the day: the window's gradual transition from darkness to light in the small hours of the morning, the first ray of sun shining in my room, the fall of the evening and the stillness of the night.

I hear the church clock chiming once and wonder if it is half past two or half past three. Half an hour later I hear a single chime. I know that it must be half past one. After lying awake another half hour, a chime rolls over the slumbering suburb: the distance toward the breaking dawn is prolonged by yet another half hour. The memory from such a night may be

34

unpleasant. Yet the night has been alive, a willful but familiar friend. I can trust these things and they are dear to me.

And I know the rhythm of the year once more. I am one with the hot silence of a summer afternoon and the persistent buzz of an incorrigible fly. The first buds on the willow and the shooting aloes are experiences leading without effort to deep gratitude.

I had forgotten that the experience of these ever-present patterns are always anchored in the incidental trivialities of the past:

> I say Mother. And my thoughts are of you, oh, House.
> House of the lovely dark summers of my childhood.*

These lines merge the image of mother and the image of house, dominant themes that bewitch me now as they have always done. For come what may, my house helps me say, I *will* be an inhabitant of the world in spite of everything. Without a house to protect us from the storms of heaven and from those of life, we would be dispersed beings.

The house to which I was brought a few days after my birth is engraved within me. It has become a complex of organic habits. After forty years, regardless of all the other anonymous steps, I can still recapture my reflex of that one high step, the step upon which as a toddler I refused to set my foot to reach my mother above; the step which harboured, tight along its riser, the slithering coil which reared its flattened head and fixed me with its beady eyes.

First and foremost, a house is a geometrical object, formed from solids and dominated by straight lines, an integral part of our carpentered world. It is a vertical being, rising upward. In middle childhood my family moved into one where the verticality was reinforced by the polarity of cellar and attic. I went down to the damp depths and up to the bright sun-trap. Years later, driving in New York City, I compared my mental house with the superimposed boxes. Lying flat on the back seat of a Cadillac™, I scanned rooms piled one on top of the other from down in the street up to their peak. But the height was purely

---

*O. V. de Milosz.

exterior; it had nothing of the personal value of verticality.

That year, as autumn gave way to the oldest of seasons, I knew the greater intimacy of a house when it is besieged by winter. After ten years, I still miss the sensation. At the time, Bill and I were both students and had no money, and not much to eat, but the house felt warm because the dark curtains made the snow beyond seem whiter and colder. With winter and its freezing temperature the house became more desirable as a place to live in. At the same time, the dialogue between house and universe was simplified. Snow reduced the exterior world to nothing. It concealed the blemishes of an inegalitarian society; it rendered us equal. You could not remark the splendour of my house, and I could not be dismayed by the decrepitude of yours. The winter cosmos is kind, comfortable; snow gives a single colour to everything and muffles every sound.

The changing seasons are imprinted indelibly on my memory. So, too, did that town which has no houses, whose skyline is made up neither of buildings nor of trees, but of signs. But what signs. They tower . . . they revolve . . . they oscillate . . . they soar in shapes which reduce the vocabulary of art history to a faculty joke. Tom Wolfe has tried to supply names: Boomerang Modern, Palette Curvilinear, Flash Gordon Ming Alert Spiral, McDonald's Hamburger Parabola, Mint Casino Eliptical. And what colours. All the new electrochemical pastels: tangerine, boiling magenta, livid pink, incarnadine, fuchsia demure, Congo ruby, methyl green, viridine, phenosafmarine, scarlet fever purple, tessilated bronze, hospital fruit basket orange.

The Baroque modern forms make Reno one of the few architecturally unified cities of the world; the style is, as Wolfe says, Late American Rich. These are the new landmarks of America, the new guideposts, the new way Americans get their bearings. They certainly gave us ours. We arrived at midnight, when everything was happening. The slot machines sounding like a cash register before the bell rings, the pictures clattering up from left to right, oranges, lemons, plums, cherries, bells. The noise churning up again and again, all over the place — that and the spins of the wheels of fortune.

The next day we woke late. Bill flung up the window blind. He turned to me slowly, face screwed up.

"Christ. It's worse than Beaufort West."

There is no home for a heart in the elaborate twists and embroidered curlicues of a skeletal sign.

Multiple sclerosis has given back to me that remarkable sense some people — and all young children — have of understanding the language of lifeless objects, and for this I am deeply grateful. I know perfectly well what generalisation and abstraction, classification and categorisation have gained for rational man: how these modes of thought have helped us control matter and energy; create man-made environments and organise ever larger social entities. The abstract, ordering intellect has added a certain majesty to our perceptions of ourselves and of the world. It was precisely the intensive study of this marvellous function of man which absorbed me completely for so many years.

Throughout the course of civilisation, those capable of the highest abstraction have often been the most humane. But abstraction also exists apart from superior intellect or humane purpose. Objective thought prepares people in our culture for what we call success; it also paves the way for mass murder. Abstraction and generalisation tend to precede territorial warfare and genocide in social evolution. How else can the State persuade teenage boys to enter Angola, unless to fight the "enemy?"

We have a word, animism, for the idea that all objects possess life. Having defined the belief, we scathingly dismiss it. Jean Piaget, the Swiss psychologist whose work has influenced me so strongly, devoted much time to its study among the children of his culture. In questioning them Piaget writes, "It is naturally necessary, and this is the most important part of the experiment, to ask "Why?" and "Why not?" after each answer." But the repeated use of "Why?" with young children is one of our most effective ways of ensuring that they do not endow the inanimate with vital force. Piaget was testing the children for animism and simultaneously influencing them against it. For there are no real whys in nature, and the hows are strictly provisional. The barrage of "whys" we bombard children with helps mould our own brand of objective consciousness — this brand of thinking built of little boxes, superimposed, tightly packed with schedules and rulers and clocks, capable of dissecting and measuring, skilled in a simple arithmetic of life and love.

The years have passed and we have observed Piaget's excellent work in practice. The filmed laboratory demonstrations are classic: the scientific-authoritative atmosphere, the white laboratory coats, the yardsticks and beakers and scales. And the bewildered little child, eyes darting around as he tries desperately to come up with an answer, any answer, that will please the avuncular man in the white coat.

At the end of the fascinating commentary we must agree with the man who has managed to dethrone King Rat. The child does indeed fail to see himself as objective and separate from nature, he does imbue things with life and he is pretty poor at abstraction, conceptualisation and all the other important things, cognitively speaking. What is more, this confusion seems to be the child's way for at least the first seven or eight years of his life.

Each generation uses its children to its own ends, Otto Rank once claimed, but so far, animistic thinking has kept us from slotting our children productively into industrialised society. We have expended time and ingenuity and money, but in this we have not yet succeeded. Nature has surely made a monumental error in creating a child who compulsively spends so much of his time fantasizing and playing.

Only when I became a nursery school teacher did I begin to realise how much the contemporary concern with the human intellect has cost us. Later I read without surprise the results of Ernest Hilgard's search for those properties of the mind that enable one person to enter a trance, that precious manifestation of the animistic mode of mind, and another not.

The kind of grown person who can alter his relationship to reality is the one who retains pleasant recollections of earlier disengagements. As a child he shared in imaginative ventures with his parents. They read to him a great deal, accompanying him on the incredible journey inward, the inner space travel that reading brings about. Or his parents told him tales, ghostly stories; together they visited giant castles in the clouds and the magic land of make-believe, played let's pretend. And, then, at the end of each adventure they brought him back — "Enough of that now, back we go," back to the world of flesh and blood people, of warm security.

For such a child the gateway between the animistic and the objective becomes a well-trodden path, a door swinging easily to and fro through which access is swift and safe. For such a child tomorrow holds fewer fears, less sorrow. Because for such a child there is the possibility later of deep religious experiences, of empathy, compassion, the ability to recognise other alternatives — all marks of a flexible tolerance impervious to the ravages of strangeness.

And so as the lifeless world comes back to life with the progression of multiple sclerosis, the abstract and the general gradually loose their hypnotic power over my perceptions. I am acutely aware of infinite possibilities long concealed by the congealing mind. New visions abound, unfamiliar intensities of feeling and being, and a delicious sensitivity to what is live, particular, unique. When things are reborn, as the willow against the white wall, or the vine over the pergola, our perceptions are finer and more brilliant. Today my room, my study, my window, my view are a world full of absorbing and breathtaking events. The diseased body is still a condition, now, at last for peace of mind. An existence devoid of sickness lacks the essential stimulus to live. The best guarantee of an unhealthy life is perfect health.

With incredible clarity now I can recall the granaries of the past, and this is suddenly an urgent incentive to me to carry on and work. As a multiple sclerotic I have found my brave new world.

If I were to go with a Trobriander to a garden where the taytu, a species of yam, had just been harvested, I would come back and tell you: "There are good taytu there; just the right degree of ripeness, large and perfectly shaped; not a blight to be seen, not one rotten spot; nicely rounded at the tips, with no spiky points; all first-run harvesting, no second gleanings." The Trobriander would come back and say "Taytu"; and he would have said all that I did and more.

Even the phrase "There are taytu" would represent a tautology, since existence is implied in being — And all the attributes, even if [the Trobriander] could find words for them at hand in his own langauge, would have been tautological, since the concept of taytu contains them all. In fact, if one of these were absent, the object would not have been a taytu. Such a tuber, if it is not at the proper harvesting ripeness, is a bwanawa; if overripe, spent, it is not a spent taytu but something else, a yowana. If it is blighted it is a nuunokuna. If it has a rotten patch, it is a taboula; if mis-shapen it is an usasu; if perfect in shape but small, it is a yogogu. If the tuber, whatever its shape or condition, is a post-harvest gleaning, it is an ulumadala. When the spent tuber, the yowana, sends its shoots underground, as we would put it, it is not a yowana with shoots, but a silisata. When new tubers have formed on these shoots, it is not a silisata but a gadena. An object cannot change an attribute and retain its identity.

—Dorothy Lee, *Freedom and Culture*. Englewood Cliffs,
   Prentice-Hall, 1959.

Being multiple sclerotic

In being in-place I am both significantly immersed in life and, at the same time, *free* of certain ways of living, widespread in our society, which are hostile to growth. I am free of experiencing life as a *race* in which I am concerned with how I compare with others: whether they are ahead or behind me; whether I am catching up to them, maintaining my distance from them, or falling behind them. Since I am not in the race, I am not caught up in the humiliation and the vindictiveness that are so much a part of the race. Also, I am free of experiencing life as a *market place* in which I see myself and others as commodities to be sold, and try to make myself into the package that happens to be in demand at a particular time. I do not experience the impotence that comes with having my sense of identity depend basically on the opinions of others instead of on the use of my own powers. Also, I am free of the *discontinuity* and chaos of experiencing life as a mere succession of disconnected events, each unrelated to what went before and what is to come. When Life is felt to be made up of unrelated fragments, there can be no appreciation of growing and maturing, and of working out or through something.

Milton Mayeroff[51]

THE terrors of suffering, sickness and death, of losing myself and losing the world, are the most elemental and intense that I know. So too is my dream of recovery and rebirth, of being wonderfully restored to myself and the world. Thus health and disease are alive and dynamic, but their modes of being are antithetical: they confront one another in perpetual hostility.

Health is an allusion to the greatest possible richness of relationship. It is a design that is infinite and expansive, reaching out to be filled with the fullness of the world. Disease is finite, endeavouring to reduce the world to itself. It is parasitic on health and life and reality. It devours the grounds of the real self. Disease and health fight to possess me, to dispossess each other and to perpetuate themselves.

Being multiple sclerotic is a complex drama enacting the reciprocity between real and false being. The plot unfolds through many distortions of time and space. It is a scenario where acts and intermissions give way to an uneven series of relapses and remissions. Multiple sclerosis may suddenly emerge from a virtual condition if I become ill, in some other way, or exhausted or shocked or depressed. The disease takes over and flourishes as health wanes. Then it may go away again, retreat into latency, with the return of strength and health.

Now others insist that there is nothing wrong with me. Even the well-intentioned persist in denying that I am ill at all. Those close to me feel an uncomfortable need to defend the diagnosis, to repeat details over and over again. It is a period of excruciating uncertainty, exacerbated by doubts and by hope, because no one can say how long remission may last — months, years or only a few days. For the disease is still there and will again come to the fore if my real being is somehow injured or lost.

Descent into relapse, once under way, proceeds by itself, gaining impetus from vicious circles, feedbacks, chain reactions: a first strain causing other strains, a first breakdown other breakdowns, with the dynamism and ingenuity peculiar to multiple sclerosis. In this curious spiral, my need for disease is joined with my susceptibility to it. Multiple sclerosis is the main part of my life now. Its sudden removal leaves a gap, an existential vacuum, that must be filled with real living if pathologic activity is not to be sucked back in to fill it.

My actions and feelings are everywhere entwined with the human and nonhuman environment as I strive for cooperation between them to realise the ultimate: remission. My weapons are the same ones I used before I became multiple sclerotic: common sense, forethought, caution and care; special vigilance and wiles to combat special dangers; and the full acceptance of what must be accepted, what cannot be changed. I have learned not to make futile attempts to transcend the possible, to deny its limits and seek the impossible. Remission does not come of itself, easily and effortlessly. It is worked for, with infinite trouble and effort, a difficult accomplishment of wide negotiation.

Remission materialises the potentialities of well-being that survive the loss of much of life and structure, as well as long immersion in illness. Being multiple sclerotic I have the mysterious capacity for health and profound disease. But remission can only be achieved and continue, if it is compatible with the totality of my relationships with the world. Unless there is harmony of being-in-relation, the state is disallowed and replaced.

Above all, it depends on maintaining proper relations with other human beings. Real being inheres in those with my husband, my family, my friends. Experiencing the fullness of the world depends on feeling the fullness of another person, as a person. Reality is given to me by the reality of people; it is taken from me by the unreality of unpeople. A look may snatch my body from me, dishearteningly estrange me from it. When I see a glance as a sneer, things around me wilt and shrivel, colours fade, light dims: my body decays a little bit more. I do not want to inhabit this body, made so alien by that other.

But when I am with a friend who shows how much she appreciates my look, my face, my body, her warmth frees me to speak as I wish, enthusiastically, now moving and shaping my body fully within the limits set by being multiple sclerotic. When I see a real smile in her smile the world sparkles with shapes, colours, light; my gaze is direct, my body no longer fettered. My friend is with me and our togetherness is made concrete in the thoughts we share and the things we observe.

My friend is patient with me and being present for me, gives me time and space to think and feel. She enlarges my sickroom whereas mere visitors narrow it. There is not distaste or reluctance in her presence, only a justification of my new form. Her speaking and hearing and seeing with me consolidates me and my body, effects cohesion between us. The stasis dissolves and I move with renewed freedom; without obstruction, I flow into my weakened arms, my obstinate tongue, into my failed eye. I inhabit my drooping body and I can do this because I am bound to my friend as is she to me. One good relation is my life-line, for kinship is healing; we are physicians to each other.

Because of my intimate connections with significant others, I feel in place in the world: my life is centered and integrated by their caring. But if caring is to orchestrate in this way it must also help me to use my particular gifts; it must arise from my uniqueness. Beyond this, I must care for and be patient with myself. I must give myself a chance to learn, to see and to discover who I am. If I fail to respond to my own needs to grow, I cannot take my place in the world.

Through finding and developing these relationships to form a centre around which my life is ordered, I live the meaning of my life. Thus, I could live differently, I could have different significant others — with the exception of myself, of course — and yet live the meaning of my life. How far this is possible is a matter of the resources available to me in the state of being multiple sclerotic. For some, particularly in regard to career, the others, or things, that they could really care about are very limited. With certain areas closed to them, they may well be unable to find and live the meaning of their lives. Inevitably, those frantically pursuing the meaning of life, confused about what is or would be relevant for their growth, unsure who they are, live in a world that cannot make much sense.

I care for my friends and I know that they need me. In consequence, I am in faith and this makes the world intelligible: I belong and I am uniquely needed, I understand and care for myself, and I can learn appropriately from my past. With this comes a deepened awareness of the unfathomable nature of our existence. There are some questions that cannot be answered, that simply have to be lived with. I see more clearly my own insignificance, as well as my incomparable worth, both part and parcel of being a once-and-for-all, like a fingerprint never to be repeated.

At remission, despite the massive functional and structural disturbances of my nervous system, I am suddenly and completely restored to myself. This is disconcerting. Under the circumstances, how can I be "nothing but" a psychologic awareness entirely reducible to my denuded brain? Surely my I-ness is something more — a nonphysical faculty perhaps, which derives its energy from my brain during life; but which as the essence of me, can survive the dissolution of my body and brain at death, establishing a connection with some other source of energy?

What is this identity, this self that cannot be lost? Man, unlike animals, is able not only to think: he can also become aware of his thinking. Consciousness and intelligence, as it were, turn around upon themselves. There is not merely a conscious being, but a being capable of being conscious of its consciousness; not merely a thinker, but a thinker capable of observing and studying his own thinking.

Among psychologists concern about the self has been erratic but never more trivial than at present. But the need to distinguish between a self or selves that can fall under one's own scrutiny from a pure or existential self that does the scrutinising has been recognised since the dawn of philosophic thought. This self, that-which-experiences, cannot itself ordinarily be experienced. We, or at least our conscious self as a personification of the five physical senses, can experience the level of being established by consciousness through the world impinging on us and the thoughts and memories deriving from it. We can experience the level of being constituted by our empirical self, a personification of the self-regulatory processes of the body functioning as another, inner organ of perception. We can also experience ourselves as objects, mechanical selves pushed around by chance or necessity. But in unexceptional circumstances we can only infer the "I" that experiences and unites this flux.

This subject able to say "I" directs consciousness in accordance with its own purposes; it is a master or controller, a power at a higher level than consciousness itself. When we speak of the self that does not change, therefore, my I-ness, we must mean the existential self. Such a word-label, however, is merely a "finger pointing to the moon" as E. F. Schumacher says; the moon itself remains highly mysterious.

The majority of graduates in any branch of biologic science alive today has the unshakeable conviction that "mind" and "brain" are one and the same thing. Or if not exactly so, then mind is some portion of the brain. All facts and all phenomena — even extrasensory perception — are properties of the brain. The physical world is the sole source of all we do or could know; there is no existence except in that sphere. Consequently, most of us doubt the truth of any religious or metaphysical teaching regarding such topics as immortality which imply a level or chain of being extending beyond ourselves. We think it only natural that the reasoning mind and its accretions of personal memories will go into the grave, disintegrate and vanish forever.

But even some orthodox research on human beings raises large doubts about the validity of this view. Certainly the research of Dr. Wilder Penfield, neurosurgeon and one-time director of the Montreal Neurological Institute of McGill University, does just that. In many operations Dr. Penfield permanently removed huge segments of the person's brain but still the "mind" seemed to carry on as before without any disruption of consciousness.

"Perhaps we will always be forced to visualise a spiritual element — a spiritual essence that is capable of controlling the mechanism. The machine will never fully explain man, nor mechanisms the nature of the spirit,"[68] he conjectured.

Moreover, all the protein of which we are primarily composed is renewed frequently. Liver and serum proteins are turned over every ten days; and that of lungs, brain, skin and muscles every 158 days.

"It is rather a frightening thought," Sir Charles Dodds once pondered, "that the whole of the protein in the human body is replaced in roughly 160 days."[23]

Today labelled isotopes are used as tracer molecules. The technique confirms that the process of renewal, the elaborate molecular synthesis, is continuous; this year's molecules are not the same as last years, even though I look and feel the same, more or less. Every atom and every molecule in my tissues is constantly swopping materials with its surroundings, so that after about six months there has been a complete turnover, with the new substances made out of what I eat and drink, and the air I breathe.

Nevertheless, when Dr. Penfield electrically stimulated the cortex of patients undergoing essential brain operations under a local anaesthetic, and therefore fully conscious, what did he find?

"The person relives a period of the past although he is still aware of the present. Movement goes forward again as it did in that interval of time that has now been, by chance, revived and all of the elements of his previous consciousness seem to be there — sights, sounds, interpretations, emotion."[69]

But how can my brain cells store my thoughts and memories and impressions if protein is so perishable, and if, as American biologist Dr. Hudson Hoagland claims, 500 billion cells of the 60,000 billion in the human body die every day and are replaced by new ones?[39]

In the 1950s it seemed that science had found the answer — DNA, for deoxyribonucleic acid. This originates in the cell nucleus and winds itself into a double helix, like two single strings of beads twisted together, along which all the necessary information for the growth of a living being is carried.

This discovery was a biochemical triumph, but it is not the secret of life. What the Nobel winning scientists had unearthed was the mechanism for relaying information from cell to cell to its final destination. What they did not tell us is how the information gets there in the first place, or how DNA can act as a matrix that enables molecules and cells to replicate themselves. Surely a matrix, to be of any use, must be independent of, and unaffected by, whatever it shapes? And surely, if it is to conserve the pattern of ever-changing material, the matrix itself must be relatively constant? But we are told that all the cells and molecules of the body are continually being torn apart and restructured so something other than a molecule is needed to maintain their form. Moreover, how does one part serve as a matrix for the whole?

Professor Harold Saxton Burr, emeritus professor of anatomy, Yale University School of Medicine, since 1935, has conducted a search for the mysterious factor which organises inanimate material into living beings and then maintains them. He found that there are electromagnetic fields associated with all living matter, from slime moulds up to man. He calls these fields of life (L-fields). In trees the L-field shows a diurnal rhythm and a lunar rhythm; it varies with sun spot activity and with the atmospheric and geophysical electrical activity of its environment. The L-fields of seeds are related to their subsequent growth characteristics and the growth and decay of the plant is accompanied by the development and decay of the L-field.

In each of us the characteristics of the L-field are linked to temperament and to physical state. There are also rhythmical variations in our L-fields relating to how we feel. Ovulation in the female is accompanied by a marked change in the L-field. Wounds cause a change in it and healing can follow the restoration of the field. Malignancy in the ovary has been revealed by L-field measurements before any clinical sign could be observed.

"Though almost inconceivably complicated, the fields of life are of the same nature as the simpler fields known to modern physics and obedient to the same laws. Like the fields of physics, they are part of the organisation of the Universe and are influenced by the vast forces of space. Like the fields of physics, too, they have organising and directing qualities which have been revealed by many thousands of experiments.

"Organisation and direction, the direct opposite of chance, imply purpose. So the fields of life offer purely electronic, instrumental evidence that man is no accident. On the contrary, he is an integral part of the Cosmos, embedded in its all-powerful fields, subject to its inflexible laws and a participant in the destiny and purpose of the Universe."[11]

The idea that the marvels of living nature are "nothing but" complex chemistry is thereby effectively destroyed, although the organising power of L-fields remains a total mystery. Professor Burr's dethronement of chemistry and therewith also biochemistry, with its DNA myth of molecules becoming information systems, is a big step in the right direction.

"To be sure" says Professor Burr, "chemistry is of great importance, because this is the gasoline that makes the buggy go, but the chemistry of a living system does not determine the functional properties of a living system any more than changing the gas makes a Rolls Royce out of a Ford™. The chemistry provides the energy, but the electrical phenomena of the electrodynamic field determine the direction in which energy flows within the living system. Therefore, they are of prime importance in understanding the growth and development of all living things."[11]

Professor Burr's conclusion seems to be that the pattern and organisation of biologic systems come about because they possess and are controlled by L-fields. But there are no principles of biologic form and function in electromagnetism, either. What exactly electricity is has been the subject of much investigation. "Electricity" Bertrand Russell said, "is not a thing, like St. Paul's Cathedral; it is a way in which things behave. When we have told how things behave when they are electrified, and under what circumstances they are electrified, we have told all there is to tell."[71]

The tale we were told by science is that electricity has a substance aspect in that it can be regarded as a "particle-ised" charge which manifests in association with substance as, for example, the electron. It also constitutes fields of force, and it radiates or vibrates in space. What electricity does *not* have, however, is consciousness or self-awareness, those essential attributes of life; how then can electrical laws explain it? Actually they do not even hint at how electrical phenomena might relate to consciousness. Something similar obtains in neurophysiology, where research has revealed the electrical and chemical processes taking place in the brain, and accompanying aspects of consciousness such as thinking, memorising, dreaming, etc. But how electrical and chemical activities in brain cells are translated into these functions is not known. Lower order concepts drawn from the mineral world to explain phenomena of higher levels of evolution will always leave a gap. They can describe whatever the two levels have in common but they can neither describe nor explain what it is that makes the one more advanced than the other.

The life fields of Dr. Burr lie outside the visible portion of the electromagnetic spectrum, and special equipment is needed to detect them. On the other hand, there is an aura of activity around all forms of animate matter that a significant number of clairvoyants are able to perceive without artificially augmenting their senses in any way. Says Dr. Pierrakos, a New York psychiatrist, "If one could see this phenomenon around the body . . . one would perceive that human beings swim in a sea of fluid, tinged rhythmically with brilliant colours which constantly change hues, shimmer and vibrate."[67]

In the late nineteenth century, Sir William Crookes — chemist and physicist — considered the possibility of a fourth state of matter, partly on the basis of his study of psychic phenomena. This state actually exists: it is called plasma, although this physical concept is not to be confused with what biologists and doctors call cell plasma or blood plasma.

The matter of which our world is composed occurs in three states: solid, liquid and gaseous. When heated, solid ice becomes liquid water, which when evaporated turns into steam, a gas. The fourth state, physical or nonorganic plasma, resembles the gaseous state. It could not be recognised until the twentieth century, after we learned more about the structure of the atom. In this state, the atoms continue to dissolve by increasingly losing their electrons, leaving behind electrically charged particles.

When the transition from the gaseous to plasma state occurs at high temperatures, the result is "hot plasma." The plasma of the lightest chemical element, hydrogen, melts into helium in the hydrogen bomb. If the plasma state is achieved with low temperatures, the result is "cold plasma."

When the fourth state of matter was discovered, no one supposed that it existed in the human body in any form. But in 1944 the Russian biologist, Dr. V. S. Grischchenko, proposed that it also existed in biologic systems and consequently in the human body, too. For a number of years various prominent Russian scientists have toyed with the idea of a cold plasma in living organisms as the basis of life.[75] They call it biologic plasma, or bioplasma.

Today, the centre of Russian bioplasma research is Alma-

Ata, the capital of the Kazakh Republic in the northern foot-hills of the Himalayas, thirty miles from the Chinese border. In one of the many technical institutes of this modern university city, Dr. Victor Inyushin, a biologist, is at work with his team.

Until the late 1950s, few attempts were made to relate physical plasma to living matter. But a number of experiments along these lines encouraged the notion that elementary particles may form a complicated, biologically organised network or system in the living organism. Inyushin and his collaborators believe that a permanent, stable state of bioplasma is possible, and that the body is constantly radiating it.[38] In conversation with Dr. Inyushin, Dr. Thelma Moss of the University of California confirmed that he conceives of the "bioplasma body" as similar, if not identical, to the aura. The smallest particles of the bioplasma are thought to influence electrical fields, rendering them visible under high frequency photography. More recently, Dr. Inyushin has tried to establish bioplasmic radiation without the use of electrical fields.

Independently of the Alma-Ata group the Leningrad biophysicist, mathematician and neurophysiologist, Dr. Sergeyev also discovered the principle of bioplasma. He started from entirely different presuppositions, developed a different instrument, and concluded that the phenomena he had observed were best explained by the assumption of the existence of cold plasma in the brain.[86,89]

Dr. Sergeyev also arrived at the view that the body radiates bioplasma. When the neurons in the brain are simultaneously stimulated according to a specific pattern, what Sergeyev calls the "biolaser effect" appears; that is, bioplasma seems to leave the brain in bundles, like photons in a laser beam. The bioplasmic ray can attain such a degree of fluctuating electrostatic charges that small objects can be moved by it.[87, 88]

Bioplasma may be a variant of plasma — or is it a fifth type of matter? In any event, biologic plasma, as distinguished from the nonorganic plasma, is a structurally organised system of free electrons and protons and the chaotic thermal randomisation force is reduced to a minimum; that is, the entropy is minimal.

The idea of a fourth state of aggregation in living organisms — possibly together with further free elementary particles — is as revolutionary (and as abstruse) as quantum physics. Nothing of it can be found between the covers of any Western medical text. The physician's concepts of the human body have not advanced beyond the formulations of nineteenth century physics and chemistry, and how many times have we been told that these were long ago displaced by the impossible possibilities of microphysics? If nothing else does, *that* certainly shows that things are seldom what they seem.

The physical world grows "curiouser and curiouser," but medicine pursues its arcane course undeterred. It can ignore these changes as easily as the evidence gathered earlier this century by men — among them physicist Sir Oliver Lodge and French physiologist Charles Richet who won the Nobel prize in 1913 — who investigated under stringent controls that strange form of matter now called bioplasma, as a fundamental constituent of the human being. In consequence, does modern medical science offer an accurate reflection of man's true physical reality?

If the theories of the Russian bioplasma researchers are verified their discoveries will radically transform our basic image of man composed over the past 200 years. We will have to take account of the fact that all living beings radiate bioplasma which, crudely, can be defined as a circulating system of electric-like waves. This becomes a field of force wherein thoughts and feelings operate in magnetic circuits, the latter appearing psychologically as so many different "me's," depending on which circuit is used by consciousness. The form and intensity of the bioplasmic radiation depends on the person's state of health, fatigue, excitement, balance, etc. It seems most strongly concentrated in the brain, although the Soviet researchers have noted particularly strong radiations from the fingers and solar plexus. In consequence, medicine will be forced to adopt new concepts for a new age, when even the fundamental electron is nothing more than a disembodied charge of energy.

Turning back to the early years of this century, the late

Walter B. Cannon, Professor of Physiology at Harvard University Medical School, pioneered studies into the workings of the autonomic nervous system, those nerves which control automatic functions, including digestion, sweating and heartbeat. In short, Cannon studied the relation of the autonomic system to the self-regulation of physiologic processes which, until the recent work on biofeedback, were thought to be outside the scope of will power or beyond conscious control by the mind.

He did much of the early work on adrenalin, the "fight or flight" hormone produced by the adrenal glands. In response to the emotions of fear and anger, adrenalin is poured into the bloodstream and carried to every part of the body in a few seconds as a chemical messenger preparing it for immediate violent action.

Adrenalin makes the heart beat faster, diverts blood from the skin and the bowels to the limb muscles and the brain, dilates the pupils and causes the muscles surrounding the bronchial tubes to relax and let more air into the lungs: all useful preparation for a fight or flight for life.

Cannon coined the word homeostasis* to mean the steady, normal state of the body maintained by the combined actions of adrenalin, the autonomic nervous system and the other adaptive processes which he studied. Not much was known in his day about the main adaptive hormone, cortisone.

He, too, was fascinated by the paradox of a body composed of soft, perishable materials, yet able to maintain a constant and almost unchanging identity for seventy to eighty years. He put it this way: "When we consider the extreme instability of our bodily structure, its readiness for disturbance by the slightest application of external forces and the rapid onset of its decomposition as soon as favouring circumstances are withdrawn, its persistence through many decades seems almost a miracle. The wonder increases when we realise that the system is open, engaging in free exchange with the outer world, and that the structure itself is not permanent but is being continuously broken down by the wear and tear of action, and as

*(from the Greek, Homeo = the same; stasis = staying)

continuously built up again by processes of repair."[14]

The ability of living beings to maintain their own constancy has long impressed biologists. The idea that disease is cured by the healing power of nature, a *vis medicatrix naturae,* was held by Hippocrates. This implies the existence of agencies which are ready to operate correctively when our normal state is upset. Much later, in 1877, the German physiologist, Pflüger, recognised the natural adjustments leading to the maintenance of a steady state when he laid down the dictum: "The cause of every need of a living being is also the cause of the satisfaction of the need."[70] Similarly, Léon Fredericq, the Belgian physiologist declared, "The living being is an agency of such sort that each disturbing influence induces by itself the calling forth of compensatory activity to neutralise or repair the disturbance. The higher in the scale of living beings, the more numerous, the more perfect and the more complicated do these regulatory agencies become. They tend to free the organism completely from the unfavourable influences and changes occurring in the environment."[28]

Again, in 1900, the French physiologist, Charles Richet emphasized this remarkable fact. "The living being is stable," he wrote. "It must be so in order not to be destroyed, dissolved or disintegrated by the colossal forces, often adverse, which surround it. By an apparent contradiction it maintains its stability only if it is excitable and capable of modifying itself according to external stimuli and adjusting its response to the stimulation. In a sense it is stable because it is modifiable — the slight instability is the necessary condition for the true stability of the organism,"[76] much as disease is the essential condition for health.

Here, then, is a truly incredible phenomenon. We are composed of material characterised by the utmost inconstancy and unsteadiness, and yet somehow we are able to maintain constancy and keep steady in the presence of conditions which might reasonably be expected to prove profoundly disturbing. The perfection we are able to attain in this regard is, indeed a miracle, particulary in the light of the work of Dr. Penfield and neuropsychologist Karl Lashley. These show that the self is not localisable, that it cannot be equated with any given brain centre or body system. It is equivalent to the intricate totality of the whole person; in his ever-changing, continuously modulated, expansive and contractive relations with the world. Their work shows, as multiple sclerosis shows, that ontologic organisation — being — unlike the yam, is a coherent entity, with an historic, stylistic and imaginative continuity. The person is not a thing-in-itself, not an organism-in-an-environment, but a being-in-relation, a being-in-an-ecosystem, a minute but active and self-aware microcosm of the world. "We see that our beings are at once unique yet communal, inherent in us, specific to us, but also in perpetual co-relation with the world: that ourselves are entelechies or monads in nature."[79]

One ancient goal of Eastern philosophy has been to establish a harmony between man and nature, to grow toward oneness. We will not be at peace with ourselves, teaches Hinduism, until we are in concert with our environment. But this is not the way of the West, particularly not at the high tide of technology and material affluence. In the philosophy of the West, nature is our most omnipresent and formidable opponent; nature exists "out there," not as a part of us but something to be possessed and mastered.

Nevertheless, the notion of universal oneness is not unfamiliar to the Western mind. In a physical sense it goes back at least 2,500 years, when Hippocrates wrote, "There is one common glow, one common breath, all things are in sympathy."[67] Other Greek sages of that era were ambitious enough to suggest the essence of this oneness. Thales of Miletus, Western civilisation's first philosopher, argued that the common wave that ripples through all matter is water. "Water" he wrote, "existed before all existing things came to be, out of which all things came and into which all things return."[67] Anaximenes claimed the universal substance was not water, but air; Xenophanes said it was earth; and for Heraclitus, it was fire. Thus came the Grecian quadruplet: earth, air, fire and water. Earth in contemporary terminology corresponds to solid matter, water to liquid, air to the gaseous state and fire to plasma.

It is no exaggeration to say that most of mankind's intellectual probings over the last 2,500 years have concentrated on finding a physical basis for universal oneness. A giant step forward came in the first decade of the 1900s. By the beginning of this century, after much reshuffling and substitution, the physical stuff of which the universe is composed had been condensed. From the Grecian quadruplet emerged two distinctly different constituents: something tangible called *matter*, and something less tangible called *energy*. All that possesses physical existence had to be one or other of these fundamental entities. And within the first decade of the century an amazing unification took place. By his celebrated formula, $E = mc^2$ (energy = mass times the square of the speed of light), Albert Einstein showed that matter and energy are interchangeable. This deceptively simple equation says that matter and energy are simply two different manifestations of a single, more fundamental entity. For lack of a better name this is called "physical existence" — not exactly the way we usually see ourselves, but accurate nonetheless.

Why did it take over twenty-five centuries to recognise the identity of matter and energy? Sir Cyril Burt's observation in his essay on "Psychology and Parapsychology" seems to provide at least a partial answer. "Our tactile perceptions of the gravitational effects of mass, e.g. a grain of sand falling on the skin, requires a stimulus of at least 0.1 gram, say about 10^{20} ergs. On the other hand, the eye in rod-vision is sensitive to less than 5 quanta of radiant energy, about 10^{-10} ergs or rather less. In detecting energy, therefore, man's perceptual apparatus, i.e. as it functions in night vision, is 10^{30} times more sensitive than it is in detecting mass. Had the perception of mass been as delicate as the perception of energy, the identity of the two would have seemed self-evident instead of paradoxical. When seeing light we should at the same time have felt the pressure of impact of the photons; and mass and energy would from the outset have been regarded as merely two different ways of perceiving the same thing . . ."[12]

Einstein's discovery was a supreme boost for the argument of physical oneness — as Banesh Hoffman says, it was a stab at "cosmic unity."[41] Now matter and energy were known to be related. Physicists turned to the next question: could one be converted to the other? The dramatic answer came on December 2, 1942, with the first sustained nuclear chain reaction. The Atomic Age was upon us.

Einstein's equation of matter and energy led inevitably to speculation about a similar equivalence between mind and matter. V. A. Firsoff, the astronomer, suggests a parallel idea. "Mind" he says, "is a universal entity or interaction of the same order as electricity or gravitation. Therefore there must exist a modulus of transformation, analogous to Einstein's famous equality $E = mc^2$, whereby mind stuff could be equated with the other entities of the physical world."[31]

The most likely place to look for such a modulus is *re-ligio*: the reconnection of man with Reality, whether this be called God, Truth, Allah, Sat-Chit-Ananda or Nirvana — the chain of being that extends upwards beyond man. Faith is the basic assumption we make about the world that leads our reason and understanding towards these sources of unknown energy.

Contact with them can be made through the self, if the "I" and the many uncoordinated "me's" can be got out of the way. To escape from them all, we must attend to Reality with "naked intent." The unwanted intruder here is thought, because it belongs to that level of being which, like multiple sclerosis, is established by consciousness; it has nothing to do with the higher levels constituted by self-awareness, a consciousness conscious of itself.

Traditional wisdom, including all the great religions, has always described itself as the Way, and given some kind of awakening as the goal. Thoughts cannot lead to a wakening to a new source of energy because the whole point is to awake from thinking into seeing with the "eye of truth." Conversely, each moment of self-awareness brings about a tiny change of direction. It may be virtually unnoticeable, but many moments of self-awareness can produce many such changes and even turn a given movement into the opposite of its previous direction. If energy is involved in these transitions it cannot be kinetic energy because as the effects of shifts in awareness, they require only a minute discharge of neuronal energy.

The self or personal identity, then, is not something we can arrive at; it is what we have to start from, an existential given in existential space. The ravages of both physical and mental diseases are superficial; there is something unfathomably deep, far beyond their reach. This is the best and strongest and most real thing we have. Once upon a time it was called the soul.

Breakdown

IT all began, I think, in 1967. That was when I first became multiple sclerotic. Now I well remember that day in late October. It was mid-afternoon when I arrived on the campus to write the first examination of the session. The large circular lawn which is the heart of the complex seemed tarnished. I glanced at my watch. 4:00 PM. Feeling quite sick, I walked listlessly into the grey shed that housed the overnight book loans. The librarian stared, eyebrows lifting slightly.

"Exam nerves?"

"I suppose so. I hope they go by 5:15. Ridiculous time, anyway, for an exam."

Whatever it was did not pass. Reluctantly I took my place in the scheduled room. Picking up the question paper, I gave a moment's thought to the time-honoured injunction to read it carefully. Dismayed, I found that I could not read it at all. I held a single sheet of paper whereon two blurred, indistinctly typed images overlapped . . . separated . . . overlapped . . . separated.

I cursed. How could I allow an exam to upset me like this? I covered my left eye but that was no good; the faint letters slithered hither and thither. I cupped my left hand over my right eye. An arm's length away I could see minute but reasonably legible bleached print. It took some time to decipher, when I picked up my pen in response. My hand shook uncontrollably. As the tip of the ball point touched the paper, my hand jerked upward across the page. That would be because of the bad pins and needles I was feeling, but it was too much. Nervous or not, I had a lot to say about the history of education. If I left the room now I would not be eligible to re-sit in January. For the next two and a half hours, I made a supreme effort. Afterwards, I had no idea which questions I had at-

60

tempted, or even how many.

Trembling, I drove to the side exit I used more than once each day. The head-lights pierced the inky night so that the road through the gate-posts was brightly lit. I stopped the car, unable to gauge the distance separating the columns. No matter how carefully I negotiated that gap I was bound to hit one or the other. My watch showed 9:00 PM before I plucked up the courage to ease the car forward.

At home, Bill was pacing the driveway. He hurried toward the car looking, somehow, larger than life.

"For heaven's sake, where have you been?"

"I've been seeing double since five o'clock, and it took almost half an hour just to get through the damned gate."

He wrenched the door open. I swung my legs sideways, grateful that the day was almost over. As my feet touched the ground, I pitched forward. Bill's outstretched hand was too late to steady me. I staggered drunkenly toward the front door. At the top of the stairs running down to our bedroom, I stopped. My legs, no firmer than jelly, would not manage the descent. Supported on each side I reached the lower landing before collapsing. Overcome by exhaustion, I was put to bed.

I woke the next morning, unrefreshed, feet numb, almost too tired to breathe. The family doctor ordered absolute quiet, bed rest and tranquilisers. Not quite a nervous breakdown, but very nearly, he thought. It would be over in a month or so; I'd certainly be well enough in January to write the examinations.

As it happened, I was still not well when the new year broke. Chronic fatigue kept me close to my bed, and I was able to walk only with great difficulty.

The four-month event was undramatic, and I was restored to full health soon afterwards, with no indication of the odd symptoms. Although I had lost an academic year, I forgot the incident and even the recurrence of an almost identical pattern toward the end of 1974 did not bring it to my mind; nor did my family recall it until much later.

Looking back to 1967 and then to 1974 and 1975 a few pieces fall into place. During these years I experienced episodes of some syndrome or disease, very similar in nature, that were severe enough in each case to incapacitate me completely for varying lengths of time. Discounting any difficulties due to the residue of iophendylate in my spine plus the excessive dosage of anticonvulsants which undoubtedly exacerbated the vertigo and fearful fits I was having toward the end of 1975, each relapse occurred in a context of considerable stress.

By the end of 1967 a few of us were seriously questioning the value of psychology to any real understanding of the human condition. We were heartily fed-up with the constant flood of verbiage we had to absorb like blotting paper, in the main a flimsy theory of learning derived from four decades of laboratory study of one or two creatures several notches down on the evolutionary scale. Nowhere is the technologic spirit or the strict pragmatism of materialism more clearly reflected than in the psychologist's ingenious emphasis on the overt response, the bar press of the pigeon, the maze running of the ubiquitous white rat and the twitches of the conditioned eyelid. The daily dunk in the font of Anglo-American psychologic wisdom was becoming tedious.

I lamented the shortcomings of psychology, Wits style, to the head of the philosophy department, weeping copiously all the while. His advice was sound: change streams or work for change in the one you have chosen. I decided on the latter course and with my rebellious soulmates poured my pent-up frustration into a new psychological journal. It was a timid venture, but drew comment in the science section of *News/Check*.

> Perhaps the most provocative article in the first issue is by Cynthia Birrer. Her point is that *all* science, in its basic form, is the study of man in his environment. Thus, in the same way that the historian uses the numismatist and archaeologist as separate but integrated authorities and allies in the same research, the psychologist should use the philosopher for the conceptualization and integration into theory of the plenitude of experimental and observed data which is at the psychologist's disposal. From this, she deduces the paradox that "philosophy and the methodology of science are beginning to stand on foundations only psychology can render secure." It is this kind of communication between separate spheres of

science that *Psychological Scene* aims to promote.[63]

It was patently clear, after the first months of the following academic year, that this reporter was the only one who was listening. We decided to have another go. I took responsibility for the second volume, canvassing contributions from England, Europe and America and coordinating them to provide a perspective on psychology, 1968. In the editorial I tried to articulate what many of us, the students, wanted to say.

> ... the Republic, despite its inhabitants' belief in the uniqueness of its position, is really a microcosm of the critical political, economic and social strains which perplex the international community. Because they inhere in the fabric of civilisation it has common problems of intergroup relations involving prejudice and exploitation. And it faces, as men everywhere must face, the most agonising question of our time: what *should be* the relation between the established, dominant white minority and the emerging masses of coloured peoples?
>
> I believe the psychologist, as a self-elected member of the empirical science committed to increasing man's understanding of man, has a responsibility to contribute more than other scientists to the ultimate solution of this problem. We all know what the relationship between white and coloured in South Africa *is* and in some limited areas the criteria and procedures of empirical science have been applied to establish what the effects of rigid separation, as defined in law, *are*. On the whole, however, the psychologist neglects both what is and what should be. For who will explore an avenue that leads only to a dead end, to utter frustration, or to exile from the land of one's birth? When it is dangerous just to think about politics, concern with the problems of the day becomes empty and futile. There are, instead, clear indications of a growing mental aloofness, a detachment from practical life. It is pertinent to ask ... whether or not a disproportionate number of psychologists, insisting on the utmost scientific rigour, have shunned the complexities of the intact human being and, in search of higher pecking status in the academic arena, planted their minds in biology, physiology, statistics, mathematics or methodology *per se*. And this at a time when the need for the psychologist's special knowledge and skills in

the human sphere has never been more urgent.[7]

Originally, of course, the university was an institution to educate scholars in a scientific discipline in relative seclusion from society. Indeed, the monastic order with its asceticism was an important model for the first university. Within its precincts, scholars approach reality in a methodical and detached way. In principle, they are liberated from the many pressures and responsibilities of the outside world to achieve this, subjected to intellectual asceticism for the sake of rational and analytic knowledge which serves humanity only indirectly. But we wanted existential rather than scientific, involved rather than theoretically detached, concrete rather than abstract knowledge.

The modern university's prime function is to stimulate and protect open inquiry and genuinely democratic discussion. But does it, in fact, confer on students (or faculty, as I found later) opportunities for the pursuit of knowledge in open inquiry? Certainly it has two diverse strings to its bow: academic studies and professional training. Nevertheless, is it really more than a factory producing the functionaries, managers and technocrats for tomorrow's industrial society? It readily becomes part of society's functionalism because of its need for a bureaucratic type of organisation. This is well illustrated by Clark Kerr's version of the multiuniversity which advocates surrender to the principles of technologic society.

Constructive protest against this orientation means finding, as in every other aspect of human life, some balance between detachment and involvement. Instead there is usually a polarisation: the professor who is paralysed by the bureaucratic-scientific attitude his position demands and cannot therefore offer existential (or relevant) knowledge confronts the student who, in giving way to his emotions, rejects the generalisations of theory and refuses to compromise with institutional realities. If there are no clear alternatives, protest inevitably becomes the goal rather than the means.

This was precisely what happened on many campuses throughout America in the sixties. But South African students are less willing to take the bit between their teeth. I concluded that editorial on a bitter note: "Subject to the insidious authoritarianism of the academic will, how quickly we learn to accept that the deeper questions of personal purpose are not worth asking and that the risks of intellectual freedom, passion and unorthodoxy are not worth taking. How soon our ideas become narrow and cautious, our thinking constrained and intolerant. How difficult it becomes to write about literature or history or religion or politics, about ethics or aesthetics, in direct, non-technical terms. As we strive for membership in the professional community we are increasingly alienated from our own feelings, intuitions and sense of relevance. If, in addition, we lose the capacity for perspective and innovation, if we relinquish our grasp of the time and culture in which we live or if our critique of the inarticulate degenerates, as has that of the hippies, into a crasser inarticulateness, and we deny the bond that binds man to man, we too will be eligible for the ranks of the withdrawn ones — the *idiotes*."[7]

By the end of 1968 I had been a student at the University of the Witwatersrand for three of my more mature years, a statement that probably means nothing to someone who has never served such a stretch. My closest friend throughout these years, Eve, and I used to sniff the air. How oppressive! How depressing! Nothing else like it in the world. We spent hours talking about it. But the confidences we shared were not sufficiently cathartic, apparently. When the doctor insisted that I was verging on a nervous breakdown, I believed him. There were plenty of reasons which had nothing to do with exam nerves why I should have come unstuck.

A year later, realising what toll my life-style was exacting, I completed a post-graduate diploma in nursery school education. I breathed the fragrance of the delightful surroundings and entered fully into the uninhibited living of the children. The contrast was vivid and I enjoyed every minute I spent in that revealing human laboratory. Obviously, though, I had not yet learned my lesson. I missed the challenge of academia and returned to university, hoping to find in education the rich contact with people which, in psychology, is conspicuous by its absence. One more degree — I had an acute dose of the diploma disease — and I joined the staff of the faculty as a junior lecturer, a situation which rapidly revealed itself to be a disastrous echo of my student days.

I stuck to it, though, twisting, compromising, stifling my real being. "Never mind," people urged when I blurted out my dissatisfactions, "Its got *status*; that's important. You can't do anything on your own these days." If you prefer quantity to quality, they were certainly right. I did not, but neither did I have the guts to quit. I tried to make the most of it, eeking out as much personal satisfaction as possible. But increasingly the cloistered' environment was sick-making, as increasingly the wider social scene that contained it was sick-making; and so like a well-conditioned rat, I made the appropriate response: I became sick, so sick that I would soon have days and months to do little but reflect on what was and what, perhaps, might have been.

I pondered the whole situation. The majority of people in any industrialised society are stressed, some more than others, and yet the majority of people do not become multiple sclerotic. It dawned on me quite slowly that even when I was maximally stressed, I succumbed each time only around the year end. Could there be any connection?

Breakthrough?*

I.

FOR the past twenty years or so I have been
the victim of virulent attacks of hayfever from September until
around April of the following year. Sneezing endlessly, eyes
pink and nose streaming, I struggle for hours on end to force
air through my blocked nasal passages, itching and scratching
until face, arms, legs, are a mass of angry raw bumps. As a
child, by the end of each day I was covered from head to toe by
repeated applications of calomile lotion.

Whenever I remember, desensitisation procedures are begun
in September and usually these alleviate the severity of the
attacks. Otherwise I rely on a huge intake of antihistamines of
one sort or another — a class of drug used to control the symptoms of hayfever and other allergies — but even so there are
many nights when I am forced to try to snatch a few hours'
sleep sitting bolt upright in bed, or a chair. For a few years
when the attacks were particularly bad, I inhaled throughout
the night the fumes of pure ammonia and this made breathing
a little easier. The attacks are always more severe after sunset.

However, the current inconveniences of this wretched condition are minor compared to the havoc wrought by the violent
allergies I developed as a child to dozens of apparently unrelated foods. No sooner had we identified paw paw as the offender and eliminated it from my diet, than another unsuspected item became intolerable. Nor were these allergic assaults
periodic. They struck suddenly, savagely, persisting relent-

*This theory is derived from the combined works of Professor W. R. Russell, formerly
Professor of Clinical Neurology, Oxford University; Professor Hans Selye, University of
Montreal; Dr. Theron G. Randolph, Chicago; and Dr. Richard Mackarness,
Basingstoke, England.

lessly until the villain had been unmasked. Somewhere along the years, in my teens I think, I outgrew the worst of it, but the allergic tendency remains, manifesting itself unmistakably, as the end of each year comes around. At present I can control matters to a limited extent by avoiding the stone fruits available in such abundance at this time.

I am never more miserable than when stricken by a bad attack of hayfever, but I have always felt too embarrassed to complain about or even to discuss it much. To the lucky ones who have never been allergic to anything — at least, that they know of — it seems too paltry to make a fuss about. So I swallow my pills, contemplate the advantages of a major share-holding in Kleenex™, and shut up.

My peculiar signs and symptoms during the past three years that, after so much pain, led to the diagnosis of multiple sclerosis have made me acutely aware that psychologists are not the only ones who have fled in the face of the intricacy of the intact human being. Sir James Mackenzie (1853-1925), one of the greatest clinicians of all time, admitted towards the end of his life that in three out of four cases he was unable to make a diagnosis. Warning against the complexities brought about by extensive specialisation in medicine, Mackenzie wrote: "For the intelligent practice of medicine and the understanding of disease, the simplification of medicine is necessary . . . I hold the view that the phenomena which at present are so difficult of comprehension on account of their number and diversity are all produced in a few simple ways, and that with their recognition what is now so complex and difficult will become simplified and easy to understand."[61]

Today multiple sclerosis is regarded as the great mystery disease, and with each new publication the mystery seems to deepen. If the veil is to be lifted on it, perhaps we should pay close heed to Sir James's words. The question is, what precipitates the multiple sclerotic plaque in those who are vulnerable? These MS types form only a small proportion of the community as a whole (1 in 1,200 in the United Kingdom; 1 in 500 in the United States).

In some respects, this problem is comparable to that of hayfever, for in this condition a small group of people are made ill by something in the atmosphere which has little or no effect on others. We know that in hayfever the cause is the presence of pollens in the atmosphere, and it now seems likely that in multiple sclerosis there must also be a factor(s) to which vast numbers of people are exposed without harm, and yet it is responsible for the multiple sclerotic plaque in those who are susceptible.

This factor(s) must be identified or defined as soon as possible, for it is likely that, whatever it is, it will be one from which the MS-prone can be successfully protected. Among those now known to precipitate demyelination are material physical injury; exposure to small domestic animals; chemicals — it has been estimated that approximately 40,000 adults suffered from polyneuritis, a demyelinating disease, as a result of thalidomide;[91] and inoculations. In this regard, Drs. Stewart and Wilson report on the incidence of brain damage (also caused by a demyelinating disease) in over 200 children, "where it seems to us impossible to explain this damage except as a consequence of the injection of the whooping cough (pertussis) component of triple vaccine (DPT) or of pertussis vaccine given by itself."[95] Infants who are not feeding well, or who suffer from allergy such as eczema or nettle rash, have been identified by Dr. Stewart as high-risk.

What do these, and other, dissimilar factors have in common? On the face of it, little if anything. Going a bit deeper, however, they can, without equivocation, be designated as stressors. (In physics a stressor exerts stress on an object in which it produces strain. The same terminology seems applicable to psychology and physiology.) Stress, in scientific terms, is the wear and tear induced in the body by the adaptive, day-to-day struggle of the person to retain her integrity and constancy in the face of potentially harmful agents, including physical and psychologic stressors of all kinds, from bad food and noisy neighbours to police brutality and fascist politics.

When environmental changes were slow and naturally occurring we responded through biologic evolution. Today they are of such magnitude and rapidity that they seriously challenge

our adaptive ability. Thus our capacity to maintain an internal
homeostasis despite changing external forces is largely oriented
to the *past*. In other words, the regulatory mechanisms identified by Walter Cannon, among others, which govern homeostasis are genetically linked to a period in our evolution quite
unlike the present. Whatever adaptability we have to ecologic
upsets was shaped by past environmental circumstances. The
catastrophic strains of industrial society and the proliferation
of new materials associated with our unprecedented affluence
constitute stressors which provoke unique responses from us.
These are a physiologic, morphologic, behavioral and social
admix whereby we seek to adapt, maintain or regain homeostatic compatibility.

In point of fact through culture, and in particular technology, we have created an environment to which we no longer
have an appropriate degree of fitness. Recently we were forced
to recognise that there are limits to overall growth as well as
more circumscribed areas of scientific advance, such as medicine; now, it seems, we have reached the limit of man's capacity
for environmental change. We do not know all the circumstances under which our ability to adapt is, or can be, pushed
beyond the point of no return. But we can expect to see, with
growing diversity and frequency, the terrifying results when we
are called upon to adapt.

Professor Hans Selye is a pioneer of modern physiologic
research into stress. He has examined numerous diseases of
organs and systems of organs, concluding that many are "diseases of adaptation," a statement which is, of course, a contradiction in terms. In these instances, the person is *not* better
adapted; rather the critical level of stability is exceeded and she
is injured instead.

Paradoxically, the mechanisms implicated by Selye in disease
are precisely those that Walter Cannon called homeostatic and
which under appropriate circumstances tend toward a stable
physiologic condition. As Cannon indicated, the homeostatic
mechanisms are clearly self-preservative. Yet, in another profound sense, Selye has shown that these very same mechanisms
are also associated with disease and death. Thus, the mecha-

nisms that are self-preservative on one occasion can be self-injurious on another.

Selye put it this way: ". . . if a dirty splinter of wood gets under your skin, the tissues around it swell up and become inflamed. You develop a boil or an abscess. This is a useful healthy response, because the tissues forming the wall of this boil represent a barricade which prevents any further spread throughout the body of microbes or poisons that may have been introduced with the splinter.

"But sometimes the body's reactions are excessive and quite out of proportion to the fundamentally innocuous irritation to which it was exposed. Here, an excessive response, say, in the shape of inflammation, may actually be the main cause of what we experience as disease . . . Could, for instance, the excessive production of a proinflammatory hormone, in response to some mild local irritation, result in the production of a disproportionately intensive inflammation, which hurts more than it helps? Could such an adaptive endocrine response become so intense that the resulting hormone excess would damage organs in distant parts of the body, far from the original site of injury, in parts which could not have been affected by any direct action of the external disease-producing agent?"[84]

The import of Selye's work is that *defense* is the key to understanding disease: it is the defensive reactions to an external agent, rather than the external agent itself (physical or psychologic) that is the nucleus of disease. In short, it is the defensive response itself that is the real and dangerous disease and this response is immanent in the individual.

In 1936, Selye published an historic letter in *Nature,* clarifying the mechanics of *general* adaptation and the body's response to the threats to its stability. It began: "Experiments on rats show that if the organism is severely damaged by acute, nonspecific noxious agents such as exposure to cold, surgical injury, excessive muscular exercise or intoxications with sublethal doses of diverse drugs, a typical syndrome appears, the symptoms of which are independent of the nature of the damaging agent or the pharmacological type of drug employed, and represent rather a response to damage as such."[83]

He went on to describe the three stages of the syndrome he had observed in his rats: Stage I comes on six to forty-eight hours after the initial injury. It is characterised by fall in body temperature, loss of muscle tone, low blood pressure, shrinking of the adrenal glands (as they squeeze as much cortisone as possible into the bloodstream in an effort to set things right) and leaking of fluid from the small blood vessels into the tissues. Selye's description of Stage I corresponds, on the whole, to surgical shock.

Stage II begins forty-eight hours after the assault on the body's stability. The adrenals greatly enlarge, the oedema or swelling of the tissues begins to subside and cell division ceases. The pituitary, the master gland situated at the base of the brain, produces increased quantities of adrenal-cortex-stimulating hormone (ACTH). When the noxious agent continues to be applied in sublethal doses, either as small repeated injuries or as small repeated doses of an allergen or harmful agent; then the rats build up resistance, become adapted to the stress, and apparently return to normal.

At this stage in his experiments, Selye, who was using cold as the stress, tried taking some of his rats out of the cold cage and putting them back into a warm environment before re-exposing them to cold. He found that they had lost their powers of resistance and had to undergo the shock reaction of Stage I again. If he left the rats in the cold, however, they continued to adapt for a long time, apparently becoming accustomed to the stress. There seemed no reason why they should not go on indefinitely in this adapted state, once they were used to it. To his surprise, however, after some weeks in the cold, his rats began to die, one by one, long before their normal life span was reached.

They had entered Stage III, the stage of exhaustion. Stage III's symptoms were similar to those seen in Stage I, but this time there was no stage of resistance or recovery to follow, only death due to exhaustion of the adaptive processes. At post mortem Selye found the rats' adrenal glands shrunken and wasted, drained of all protective hormones and incapable of producing any more.

Explaining the significance of these three stages, Selye wrote: "We consider the first stage to be the expression of a general alarm of the organism when suddenly confronted with a critical situation, and therefore term it the "general alarm reaction." Since the syndrome as a whole seems to represent a generalised effort of the organism to adapt itself to new conditions, it might be termed the "general adaptation syndrome." It might be compared to other general defence reactions such as inflammation or the formation of immune bodies.

"The symptoms of the alarm reaction are very similar to those of histamine toxicosis or surgical or anaphylactic shock; it is therefore not unlikely that an essential part in the initiation of the syndrome is the liberation of large quantities of histamine or some similar substance, which may be released from the tissues either mechanically in surgical injury, or by other means in other cases. It seems to us that more or less pronounced forms of this three-stage reaction represent the usual response of the organism to stimuli such as temperature changes, drugs, muscular exercise, etc., to which habituation or inurement can occur."[83]

Selye has spent the last forty years studying stress. The results have led to enormous advances in medicine and psychiatry: new treatments have been developed for shock, rheumatism and anaphylaxis; and psychiatrists now have a clearer understanding of the physiologic basis for nervous breakdown.

However, since he is a physiologist and works mainly with animals, Selye has not himself applied his concepts in a clinical setting. Had he done so, he would have noted — particularly in the field of allergy — that adaptation and maladaptation show themselves more often as specific symptoms related to specific stressors and individuals, rather than as general to all noxious agents and all people. Professor Adolph, a physiologist at the University of Rochester School of Medicine, observed and reported similar stages of adaptation to those noted by Selye; but he also found that individual animals showed marked differences in their responses to the same agent, and that these responses were more often specific to a particular stress, than general to all.

Working with healthy experimental animals, Selye and Adolph exposed them to regular doses of a given harmful material, under controlled conditions, and watched them show alarm, adapt, develop illnesses in the exhaustion stage, and finally die.

The sick do not usually consult their doctors until they are entering the stage of exhaustion in their struggle to adapt to an environmental stress. Lacking a means of turning back the clock in the person's illness, the doctor is left to speculate on causes and to treat symptoms empirically as they arise.

In multiple sclerosis, particularly, there is the topsy-turvy situation of one neurologist after another mistakenly citing the symptoms as the cause of the illness. My excessive fatigue was said to be due to neurasthenia, and my pain, convulsions and increasing failure of mobility to hysteria. Instead, the entire set of symptoms, or syndrome, should have been attributed to the demyelination following the exhaustion caused by constant exposure to the stressor(s) to which I was allergic.

The word allergy (literally, other response) was coined in 1906 by Clemens von Pirquet, a Viennese paediatrician who worked on diphtheria in children with Dr. Béla Schick, originator of the Schick skin test for immunity to this disease. Von Pirquet defined allergy as an acquired, specific, altered capacity to react to physical substances on the part of the tissues of the body.

Although allergic illnesses have been recognised and described since ancient times, they are still imperfectly understood. It is known, however, that allergies to specific substances are acquired by exposure to those substances and that a general tendency to react in a hypersensitive or allergic manner is hereditary. It has been estimated that a family tendency to allergic reactions affects as much as 80 percent of the population in developed countries.

Allergy as a medical subject grew up within the framework of immunology: the study of immunity or resistance to infection by the microorganisms of smallpox, diphtheria, tetanus, typhoid and other contagious diseases. Early researchers in this field found that, in addition to the desirable immune response following the injection of dead germs (called antigens because they generate antibodies), they also encountered hypersensitivity reactions. This discovery led to the development of skin tests for immunity. These and subsequent injections form the basis of the public health immunization programs established to protect children from such infections as scarlet fever and diphtheria, which were responsible for so many deaths in the nineteenth century. However, some people become hypersensitive or allergic as well to the antigens with which they are injected.

Immunity and allergy, the two antithetical responses to inoculation with identical material, were explained by von Pirquet as *changed* reactivity following exposure: on the one hand, acquired or induced immunity; on the other, hypersensitivity. Both are based on the chemically understood antigen-antibody reaction and are demonstrable by the skin tests which have since become the *sine qua non* of orthodox allergy practice.

Convention is a powerful force in medicine, and for years now most allergists have restricted their clinical work to conditions like asthma and hayfever which do respond to skin tests and desensitizing injections with graded doses of allergens — pollens, house dust and similar inhalant antigens being amongst the most common.

Against this background of almost three-quarters of a century of conventional allergy practice, Albert Rowe in California began drawing medical attention to the importance of food allergy as a factor in many common diseases. His approach was empirical and clinical, in line with von Pirquet's original wide, biologic view of allergy.

II.

In addition to their powers of general adaptation, human beings are also capable of variable degrees of adaptation in the sense of specific and individualised responses to environmental exposures occurring in the presence of equally variable degrees of individual susceptibility. However, it is the *total* load of environmental exposures, both specific and nonspecific agents, that are important in determining whether an individual adapts (remaining relatively symptom-free) or maladapts (manifesting chronic symptoms) at any given time.

The environmental agents capable of inducing high degrees of individual susceptibility and eliciting specific, as opposed to general, adaptation have been the life-long concern of Dr. Theron G. Randolph of Chicago. His interest ranges from those considered harmless, such as the common foods studied by Rowe, to those known to be toxic in greater concentrations but alleged to be harmless in the amounts ordinarily encountered, e.g. the chemical additives to food.

Chemicals in the diet, which are eaten every day, are not suspected of causing allergic illness, even by those most alarmed at their use. Poisoning, not allergy, is what is feared. Randolph, however, says in his book, *Human Ecology and Susceptibility to the Chemical Environment,*[73] that he has found chemical additives and contaminants of air, food, water, as well as chemically derived drugs, to be a more common cause of allergy and chronic illness than the more generally recognised naturally occurring physical and biologic materials, such as unprocessed foods, animal products and plants.

He emphasized that allergy to the foods themselves and to their chemical contaminants can give rise to identical symptoms, although those associated with the latter tend to be more severe. He has demonstrated that one-third of his patients have major allergies to new materials in the chemical environment. Even gas and petrol fumes, whose allergic effect is difficult to place in terms of immunology, have been shown to affect detrimentally highly susceptible people, even in minute dosage. In fact, I had the worst allergic attacks of my life while living on the top of a high-rise building in Hillbrow, a high density area in Johannesburg; these attacks resisted every effort by the ear, nose and throat specialist either to identify or subdue. For another third of Randolph's patients such allergies, while not "major," appear to be a significant contributing factor to their problem.

Randolph cites the interesting case of a previously symptom-free woman, highly susceptible to a wide range of environmental chemical exposures but remaining well in her own engineered and controlled living quarters, who visited another home containing gas-fired utilities. A few minutes after sitting down, and quite unaware of any unusual odour, she starts first moving her feet, then shuffling the feet and legs, crossing them this way and that. Next she starts shifting her entire body, rubbing her thighs with her hands. Becoming increasingly nervous and fidgety, she gets up and walks around. At about this time her face becomes flushed and conversation becomes increasingly difficult. Her face reddens further; speech becomes disconnected, sometimes slurred; irritability and ataxia (jerkiness and clumsy motion) begin to manifest. Hyperactivity, stumbling gait, blurred vision which goes on to strabismus (cross-eyedness), puffiness and stiffness of her fingers, and then sudden physical collapse and stupor ensue. After sleeping several hours, she awakens with severe generalised muscular aching and soreness, and feeling depressed, a response sequence precipitated by an inhalation exposure(s) only.

Ecologic illness is defined as an adverse reaction to an environmental insult or excitant in air, water, food, drugs or our habitat — domiciliary, occupational or avocational. Because it is not yet recognised for what it is, no statistical studies have been made, and we can only estimate its incidence. According to Dr. Mackarness, 30 percent of people attending general practitioners have symptoms traceable exclusively to food and chemical allergy; 30 percent have symptoms partially traceable to this cause, and the remaining 40 percent have symptoms unrelated to allergy.[60] If he is right, and there is support for these figures from the United States, there is a need for a complete change in the medical approach to ill-health, and a total revision of government policy and regulations concerning food. Moreover, clinical iatrogenesis becomes a very serious matter indeed.

The stimuli that elicit the gradual dynamic modifications leading to specific adaptation are either sustained or occur intermittently, encouraging a cumulative effect. This enhances their ability to induce and maintain high degrees of individual susceptibility and, later, to manifest as advanced, unrecognised constituents of specific adaptation. Although many other environmental agents can also induce extreme degrees of individual susceptibility, in general their effect is less sustained and the forms it takes are less obscure and complex than those deriving from foods, drugs and environmental chemical exposures.

Randolph heard Selye present his new idea about the general adaptation syndrome in 1944 at an allergy society meeting, eight years after his famous letter appeared in *Nature*. But it was not until 1954, ten years later, that Randolph realised that Selye's three stages of adaptation — alarm (nonadaptive and immediately reactive), resistance (adapting), and exhaustion (again, nonadapted) — were equally applicable to specific adaptation.

In tracing the spontaneous development of a chronic ecologic illness, Randolph starts from a baseline, or level 0, considered as a position of stability and balance — homeostasis — to which we have a built-in tendency to revert.[74] Every specifically adapted response has a long-term developmental course, often starting at birth or before. All have both stimulatory and withdrawal phases that exist along a continuum extending from the two outer extremes toward the centre or homeostasis.

Like Selye's general adaptation, the specific variety also occurs in three stages. In Preadaptive Stage I, sustained nonpersonal environmental exposures in conjunction with low grade individual susceptibility might be expressed as mild delayed symptoms. Conversely, sporadic exposures to increased susceptibility are likely to produce an acute nonadapted response; the greater the degree of individual liability, the greater its immediacy and severity. From this point, however, the course followed by intermittent and cumulative exposures diverges. The former continue to trigger the violently acute reaction which everyone recognises as allergic.

Randolph subdivides Addicted Stage II into adapted and maladapted sequential phases. If repeated exposures in the presence of individual susceptibility are maintained, the immediate effects are reversed; now a specifically adapted relatively symptom-free state ensues. The initial stimulatory responses comprising this can persist for long periods of time; in fact, reactions may never develop beyond this relatively desirable level, which is often confused with normalcy, or level 0.

The absence of acute reactions is apt to be interpreted as outgrowing or tolerance of the incriminated exposure. Children known to be susceptible to a given food are often said to have outgrown their allergy. (I was.) Actually, decreased susceptibility merely indicates a move from an unmasked (non-addicted) type of response to a masked or addicted one.

The speed of reversal from the one to the other varies with the degree of individual susceptibility existing at the time. Usually the change is insidious if regular reexposures occur prior to an established susceptibility and continue as it builds up. Now the preadaptive acute reactions are either bypassed or just not recalled later. At least in the early stages of developing specific adaptation, the person is ordinarily oblivious to the spontaneous beginnings of her ecologically related disturbances. A specifically addicted person is unaware of ill effects, or she may even feel better after consuming an addicting substance.

Specifically adapted persons tend to become hyperactive and irritable when the impact of regular exposures is amplified by growing individual susceptibility to them. In general, they do not regard themselves as abnormal or ill, although this view may not be shared by their family or friends. A hyperactive salesman is unlikely to admit any difficulty as long as sales are booming and customers are satisfied. Instead he prides himself on his dynamism, only becoming concerned after he has burned himself out.

This transition from predominantly adapted to mainly maladapted responses marks the apparent onset of the current illness. It is a subtle change associated with a gradual sense of pervasive ill health, or general malaise. Burning oneself out seems to be a synonym for the switch from the initial stimulatory to the subsequent withdrawal phase of reaction.

Not uncommonly, relatively symptom-free adaptation changes to maladapted symptom-related responses during and following infections, especially virus infection. Infectious agents can produce their symptoms by increasing the number and intensity of allergic responses to foods and chemicals. Relapses in multiple sclerosis, of course, are often triggered by infections.

People rarely visit their doctors when they are well, that is, either in the preadaptive stage or when adapting and relatively symptom-free. Rather they seek medical assistance only when they can no longer cope with their illnesses. This usually happens when or shortly after the adapted stage merges with and is then superseded by maladaptation. To what and for how long the person has been adapting to one or more environmental substances is a mystery to all concerned. If there is no infection or other obvious difference in exposures to account for the present illness, the individual is unable to help her doctor uncover the cause(s) of her maladapted responses. Instead, she is at the mercy of his clinical judgment which, Sir James MacKenzie tells us, is likely to miss the mark in three cases out of four.

The most common withdrawal syndromes which follow the stimulatory phase are localised allergic manifestations. These include upper and lower respiratory tract syndromes: rhinitis, pharyngitis, laryngitis, bronchitis, asthma; eye and ear syndromes: photophobia, conjunctivitis, blurring or dimness of vision, excessive itching and lacrimination; running ears, earache, deafness and tinnitus; gastrointestinal conditions: colitis, diarrhea, constipation, nausea, vomiting; genitourinary conditions: urgency, frequency, tenesmus, proneness to urinary tract infections. Any organ system allergy tends to exhibit excessive mucus production, edema, and is often complicated by hypertrophy of reacting tissues, as well as infections. Involvements of tubular structures, such as the bronchi and genitourinary tract, sometimes lead to obstructive complications.

One or more of these localised allergies often coexists with systemic allergic syndromes. Fatigue and related behavioral disturbances were first reported in this context in 1930 by Albert Rowe.[77] Fatigue as a constitutional expression of individual susceptibility and maladaptation to specific environmental exposures is characterised by tiredness and mental torpor unrelieved by the ordinary or even an excessive amount of rest. Present to at least some degree all the time, it materially reduces initiative, wit, reading speed and comprehension.

Headache is almost equally frequent as a demonstrable specific maladapted response. Although many investigators point out that the majority of headaches meeting the classical description of migraine and other variations may be diagnosed specifically, the rarity with which this is actually attempted is startling. According to Randolph, headaches should be explored from the standpoint of their probable ecologic etiology rather than be endured or treated symptomatically. I doubt that he excluded from this maxim the migraines from which so many multiple sclerotics suffer.

Rowe also identified the allergic etiology of various muscle aches and pains as a part of the clinical picture of allergic toxemia. Allergic responses involving the skeletal musculature are usually localised to the muscles of the posterior cervical region, upper back and shoulders. Myalgia (muscular pain) of allergic origin occurs in the posterior cervical muscles, calf muscles, the hamstrings, lower muscles of the back, pectoral muscles, intercostals and the rectus abdominus, in that order. It may be a specific allergic response of striated musculature; it may involve a particular segment of a given muscle, an entire muscle, or regional groups of muscles; or it may manifest as generalised muscle soreness and aching, especially upon arising in the morning after the ingestion of allergenic foods the previous day.

More specifically, complaints of allergic myalgia range from nagging sensations of pulling, drawing, tautness and aching of involved muscles to sharply localised, severe cramp-like pains. The latter may or may not be associated with nodular areas of increased firmness and tenderness in the bellies or insertions of affected muscles. Those muscles involved commonly become gelled or more rigid during sleep so that either chronic or acute symptoms are accentuated by the first movement upon waking. Instances of acute torticollis, acute lumbago or acute bursitis are not unusual. Even less so, however, is the chronically ill person who is lame, stiff and generally sore upon getting up in the morning.

The most important point in making a tentative working diagnosis of allergic myalgia is to think of it. This possibility is rarely ever considered and even more rarely approached by means of diagnostic-therapeutic measures capable of identifying and avoiding the most common environmental incitants and perpetuants of this condition: namely, specific food addictants, environmental chemical exposures and house dust.

Chronic manifestations of allergic myalgia may present either as sustained stimulatory or withdrawal responses. The most recent description of the recurrent stimulatory phase, "restless legs," was published in 1960. An editorial in the *British Medical Journal* describes the syndrome thus: "The essential feature of the condition is an intolerable creeping, internal itching sensation, often defying description, occurring in the calves and lower legs, sometimes in the thighs, usually bilaterally and developing towards the end of the day when the patient is either seated or particularly in bed. So unpleasant is this sensation that the patient is compelled to keep moving his limbs, and this movement will bring relief."

The onset of the more painful intermittent or chronic withdrawal phase, to which the term myalgia is generally restricted, occurs only later in the developmental course of the illness. The paresthesias accompanying the restless legs syndrome sometimes merge with allergic pain syndromes, including headache, and muscle and joint aches. There comes a time apparently, when the energetics of cellular function simply cannot provide sufficient potential to maintain the stimulatory phase of allergic myalgia and one, or often more than one, of the painful allergic syndromes come to dominate the chronically ill individual.

Generally, though, the myalgia becomes so prominent that the person fails to mention that she was a hyperactive child, from which she gradually recovered. Of course, it is possible for the entire stimulatory-withdrawal sequence to occur rapidly, or at any age.

Extremes of hyperactivity could be maintained, provided the identity of the addicting substances is known to the person or there is sufficiently frequent exposure to them. In addition she must possess the ability to be stimulated, the exact bodily mechanism of which is still poorly understood. Without these requirements, advanced stimulatory levels are not apt to be sustained.

Where they are, the behavior of these euphoric individuals is often marked by an exaggerated, poorly controlled motor activity, expressed in a degree of ataxia suggesting drunkenness. Occasionally, there is excessive giggling or pathologic laughter as well as such vasomotor responses as flushing, sweating and chilling.

The more advanced withdrawal responses of ecologic origin include mild depression and disturbed mentation: confusion, forgetfulness, indecisiveness, impaired reading comprehension, aphasia, shortened attention span as well as moodiness, sullenness and slightly withdrawn and apathetic behavior. In more severe responses, depression, with various degrees of stupor, lethargy and impaired responsiveness and mental lapses, blackouts and epileptic seizures may also occur.

The chronically ill person presents alternating syndromes: on the one hand, changeable stimulatory and withdrawal levels with acute and chronic manifestations correlating, respectively, with the intermittency or chronicity of responsible environmental excitants; on the other, a wide range of interrelated physical and mental syndromes. To the doctor whose clinical acumen is stretched to its very limits, she is a mishmash of symptoms. Even his armamentarium of investigatory procedures is unable to uncover anything definite. At his wits end, so far as the doctor is concerned, the more numerous the complaints, the less the significance of any of them; the individual is nothing but a neurotic. Many chronically sick, aware of this attitude among doctors, focalise and distort their medical histories to avoid giving the impression of a raving lunatic.

The allopathic doctor notwithstanding, however, the alternation between psychologic and allergic manifestations is an oft noted phenomenon. Also, recurring swings in the levels of presenting symptoms may have an endocrine basis. Examples include women experiencing accentuated allergic pain, headaches and myalgia, and other syndromes premenstrually and, less frequently, at the time of ovulation. Exactly fourteen days before every period I am virtually incapacitated by the flare-up of the chronic burning pain at the base of my spine, across both buttocks and down to the tips of the lower extremities. The endocrine link with allergic symptoms is interesting in view of the fact that women are more frequently victims of multiple sclerosis, and that it rarely manifests before puberty or after menopause.

Randolph's final stage, or Postadapted Stage III, is similar to the preadapted one in that irrespective of the past frequency of intake, each specific reexposure is followed by an immediate acute reaction. Under these circumstances, the identity of the addictant is no longer a problem. This final stage of specific adaptation is seldom reached spontaneously.

Retrospectively, it is impossible to trace the origin of specific susceptibility and adaptation to multiple materials. There may be predisposing factors, such as biologically susceptible groups of cells with hereditary and/or nutritional defects. However, once a person becomes susceptible to a given ecologic agent, there seems to be a tendency for the process to encompass an increasingly wider range of the *milieu exterior* able to induce individual susceptibility. Initially, there is probably a restricted set of environmental offenders — particulate inhalants such as pollens, spores, dusts, insect and animal danders — to which there are lesser degrees of individual susceptibility and which tend to be present at lesser stimulatory-withdrawal levels.

Foods, biologic drugs and environmental chemical exposures may also manifest at these lower levels; however cumulative long sustained exposures to foods and environmental chemicals are especially apt to be associated with higher degrees of individual susceptibility and to be present in advanced stimulatory-withdrawal sequences. Although at first only a few agents may be incriminated, with time the allergic process embraces a progressively wider scope of environmental exposure and manifests as advanced stimulatory-withdrawal syndromes. Also with advancement of the allergic process, the more rapidly occurring and the greater the swings between levels of stimulatory and withdrawal effects. The tendency of the allergic process to spread and to advance in degree, once initiated, is known as *individualised epidemiology.*

Marked variations between individuals are to be expected. Moreover a given person may be highly susceptible to one agent and only slightly so to another. Also larger and/or more rapidly absorbed variations of a given item than that to which one is accustomed may break through specifically addicted responses and precipitate acute reactions. Someone adapted to two slices of bread per meal (or its equivalent wheat content) often finds that a spaghetti dinner, which represents two or three times her usual intake, makes her sick. A person blindly addicted to the customary intake of corn in its edible form tends to react acutely to one or two drinks of bourbon whisky.

In advanced circumstances, a multiplicity of addictive substances are usually involved in addicted responses, the combination of which manifests in chronic illness. Also addictive substances have a characteristic tendency to reinforce or to substitute for others.

In view of the vogue in many quarters to treat multiple sclerosis by means of drug therapy (including steroids and immunosuppressants) the apparent effects of this on the individual's ability to adapt is important. The net results of maintenance drug therapy for chronic illness of ecologic origin are that it increases the load to which adapation must be attempted; permits specific susceptibility to spread by means of cross-reactions to related materials; and favours the development of new susceptibilities, *including adverse reactions to the therapeutic agents employed.* Sooner or later maintenance drug therapy either leads to advanced addictive phenomena or to depletion of bodily defences, the stage of exhaustion of general adaptation.

III.

The pattern of disease has changed drastically since the Industrial Revolution began to alter our environment, particularly our diet. Coronary thrombosis, which now kills about 100,000 people annually in the United Kingdom alone, was unknown to nineteenth century physicians. Not until 1910 was the first case described in the British medical literature. Now, instead of the devastating epidemics of infectious diseases like typhoid, TB, cholera and smallpox that used to decimate us before the twentieth century, we have equally devastating epidemics of strokes, high blood pressure, heart attacks, behavioral disorders and degenerative diseases. All these have taken over, leaving us little healthier than we were 100 years ago. What is the reason?

The germ theory of disease had an enormous impact on medical science, but we think of germs alone as the enemy. This cornerstone of modern allopathic medicine states that certain microscopic entities — bacteria and viruses being most important — whose appearance in space and time correlates well with other physical manifestations of illness, are causative of illness. Therefore, the theory continues, infectious illness can profitably be treated by trying to force these entities out of existence.

One of the great contributors to this theory was the German bacteriologist and Nobel laureate, Robert Koch, whose reasoning regarding the etiologic, i.e. causative, relationship between a microorganism and a disease eventuated in Koch's Postulates: (1) The microorganism must regularly be isolated from cases of the illness. (2) It must be grown in pure culture *in vitro*. (3) When such a pure culture is inoculated into susceptible animal species, the typical disease must result. (4) From such experimentally induced disease the microorganisms must again be isolated.

In fact, fulfillment of these postulates does no more than establish a correlation between the presence of the germ in the body and the other physical manifestations of the illness as observed in animals. It does not prove that real world human beings get the same physical illness because they come into contact with the germ. You may ask, doesn't fulfillment of Postulate 3 prove cause? The animal was healthy before the germ was put into it and sick afterwards. True. But inoculating animals with germs is a grossly unnatural procedure that obscures the relevance of any subsequent observations to the world beyond the laboratory.

Experimental rigour obtained at the expense of relevance to the world at large is of questionable value, to say the least. It greatly increases the risk of formulating hypotheses that explain the data, but which are of no real use to us. We live in a world full of germs, some of which are associated with physical symptoms of infectious disease. But only some of us get infectious diseases some of the time. Why? Because there are factors *in us* that determine what kind of relationship we will have with those germs that are always out there, a relationship of balanced coexistence or one of unbalanced antagonism. Fulfillment of the third of Koch's postulates bypasses the whole system by which relationships with germs are internally determined, as Dr. Andrew Weil points out.[104] It shuns the complexities of the intact human being, the being-in-his-ecosystem, in favour of scientific precision, a specious move in *any* area of applied science.

In short, germs need the right environment in which to grow, and the tissues involved in allergic reactions make ideal seed-beds for bacteria and viruses. There has been much discussion about the possible role of a slow virus in causing multiple sclerosis. Certainly it seems likely that a virus disease affecting the nervous system in early life may lead to the immunological abnormality found in MS-vulnerable people, but it now seems very unlikely that reactivity of the former virus infection could possibly lead to the formation of so many fresh plaques in entirely new sites, a very characteristic feature of so many multiple sclerotic patterns.

Sensitivity of the nervous system may show up as neuritic pain, *tic doloureaux*, Bell's Palsy, or any one of a whole group of mental and neurologic symptoms caused by local swelling and irritation of cells in different parts of the brain. There may also be a general feeling of fatigue, possibly produced by internal swelling of specific cells. Any or all of these will be familiar to every multiple sclerotic.

We do not yet know why some people are more susceptible to allergy than others, or why the allergic target organ is the gut in one person and the nervous system in another. Professor

Russell has made one suggestion as to why the latter should be the target organ.[78]

Those who study experimentally the various ways in which the brain can be injured by allergic processes point out that it is well protected in this regard until the blood-brain barrier (BBB), a physiologic system necessary for the normal function of the brain, is breached. Attempts to localise the site of this barrier to some specific anatomic structure led finally to the conclusion that every membrane existing between blood and brain may contribute to the BBB. The brain requires an exceptionally vigorous circulation of blood during both day and night, and this is so much the case that if the circulation is rendered inadequate the brain cells begin to perish within a few minutes owing to lack of oxygen. The oxygen, glucose, etc., continually conveyed to the brain by the bloodstream pass to the brain cells from the blood capillaries. Under normal circumstances any blood cells, such as lymphocytes, are prevented from leaving these. The BBB appears to be most vulnerable at the point where the tiny capillaries join together to form minute veins, and this is the beginning of the return journey of the blood from the brain to the heart.

It is around these venules of the white matter of the brain and spinal cord that the multiple sclerotic plaques form and this happens in those regions where the circulation is most sparse. Their development around small blood vessels is the central "hard" fact relating to multiple sclerotic lesions. The first sign of a new plaque seen by the microscope is the escape of some lymphocyte from venule to brain tissue. Lymphocytes are the cells that make up our immune system. Like the nervous system, this penetrates most tissues of the body. Oddly, the two systems seem to avoid each other: the BBB prevents lymphocytes from coming into contact with nerve cells. Thus, the movement of a lymphocyte to brain tissue is a visible sign of a fault in the BBB.

The new plaques as seen in the rare autopsies of acute cases are not sclerotic; they are infiltrations by fluid of the nerve tissue surrounding blood vessels. That is, the patch is not sclerotic initially but fluid, edematous; it only becomes so later.

Conversely, the old patches are sclerosed. The agent or factor that makes the coats of these vessels permeable to serum is the crux of the matter.

Decreased capillary resistance together with increased permeability have been observed in rats on a polyunsaturated fatty acid (PUFA)-deficient diet. Capillary resistance of humans, especially in those people with allergic manifestations, was higher in people receiving vegetable oils than in those on a diet containing animal fats.

The anatomic relationship of blood vessels to small early plaques has been studied intensively since the last century. Although it has been a matter of prolonged controversy, Dr. Lumsden, a foremost researcher into multiple sclerosis, concludes that the evidence does indicate the frequent presence of a small venule in the centre of the younger and smaller lesions. He states that while venules appear to have "some influence in determining the sites of origin of the plaques, they do not determine the subsequent evolution or form of the plaque."[50]

The view that the plaque develops as the direct result of occlusion, probably due to thrombosis, has its champions as well as detractors. But recently there has been more than one suggestion that temporary occlusion of small blood vessels in the central nervous system resulting from agglutination and aggregation of blood platelets may be responsible. And, indeed, platelet stickiness is increased during exacerbations and returns to normal in the quiescent phases. This rise in degree of adhesiveness may be associated with histamine, a chemical released by the platelets in response to entry into the central nervous system of some allergen(s). The resultant clumping of the platelets causes blockage of small venules, although perhaps only of transient duration.

Since platelet stickiness presumably is widespread throughout the bloodstream as a whole why are the effects of the platelet microthrombi restricted to the central nervous system? Why are only our brains and spinal cords affected? One possible reason is that, in general, the peripheral tissues have relatively large extracellular spaces and a system of lymphatic drainage, whereas the extracellular space in the central nervous system is almost certainly small (traditionally, expanded extra-cellular space in plaque tissue is an indication of BBB insult) and the brain and spinal cord have no lymphatic system. The effects of even temporary blockage of small blood vessels are therefore likely to be greater in the central nervous system than in other tissues; also, in addition to the hypoxia following occlusion, the small extracellular space and the absence of lymphatic drainage will tend to minimise the dilution of the area of histamine, and other possibly cytotoxic compounds, released from the platelet thrombi.

If the problem of nervous system susceptibility to neurologic insult is reduced to one primarily concerning the circulation, it may be significant that countries and communities in which multiple sclerosis is common are also those in which coronary heart disease is frequent, though the problem usually affects a different age-group. Heart attacks due to coronary artery disease are not uncommon in the middle-aged person with multiple sclerosis. Migraine is also relatively common in people with multiple sclerosis.

The blood supply to the brain and spinal cord normally increases quickly during the first ten years of life, but then there is a surprising change, for although the blood supply of the nerve cells (grey matter) continues to increase during the second decade of life, the blood supply of the white matter is slowly reduced during this period, apparently due to the fact that by the age of about twelve years the myelin sheaths have acquired their full thickness and the processes of mere mainte-nance as opposed to growth make less demands on the circula-tion. Multiple sclerosis rarely appears before the age of fifteen, and it may be significant that at this age the vulnerable areas of the white matter are experiencing some reduction in their supply of blood for physiologic reasons.

In general, multiple sclerosis is less prevalent where babies have been breast fed. This fact is usually invoked to support the suggestion that nervous system susceptibility arises from faulty nutrition early in life. However, work by Drs. Hofer and Weiner point to the operation of more subtle mechanisms lending indirect support to a link between poor circulation and susceptibility to multiple sclerosis. These researchers have found that some aspect of the feeding interaction with the mother regulates cardiac sympathetic tone and respiratory rate control at relatively high levels in the newborn rat in the pre-weaning period, and that in the absence of this stimulation, these rates decline. They propose that early experience of maternal separation may affect the pup through at least two different and separate processes. "Cardiorespiratory regulation may depend on nutritional intake — rather than be determined by an innate homeostatic set point — during the experience, while acute behavioral responses may be primarily determined by some other aspect of the separation experience, presumably involving disruption of the social interaction between mother-pup."[40]

The question as to whether there are some occupations which protect the person from ever suffering from multiple sclerosis might throw some light on etiology, but this important topic has been neglected. Russell has found athletes in full training are virtually protected, whereas those who were athletes previously but abandoned their training owing to the pressure of business, etc., may become vulnerable after two or three years. On theoretical grounds, Russell suggests that heavy manual labour for forty hours a week, of almost any variety, would also give protection from the dangers of multiple sclerosis, even if the typical allergic tendency was known to be present.

On the other hand, increased susceptibility of the nervous system to neurologic insult through damage to the BBB may, in fact, have less to do with circulation than nutrition, specifically the switch from breast to bottle feeding which has transformed the traditional suckling into a modern baby. The pattern of worldwide modern malnutrition is particularly reflected in the two forms that infant malnutrition takes. The change from breast to bottle introduces Chilean babies to a life of endemic undernourishment; the same switch initiates British babies into a life of sickening, addictive overalimentation.[65]

Changing nutritional factors in infancy are generally considered in terms of their potential relationship to permanent alterations in myelin composition. The two kinds of essential fatty acids (EFAs) which man requires in his diet are linoleic and linolenic acid, and while these are present in human milk, they are absent from cow's milk. Moreover, this has a great diversity of short chain fatty acids, some of which have not been described in other dietary sources and are possibly of toxic effect. An idea which has rapidly gained popularity is that the considerable differences between human and cow's milk provide a metabolic basis for permanent alterations of brain lipids. In short, a deficiency of these EFAs during development is a factor — some think *the* factor — in the etiology of multiple sclerosis.

Slight changes in the fatty acid composition of brain lipids in multiple sclerotics have been claimed by some investigators. But although the white matter they studied did appear normal on visual inspection, it may well have contained small or early demyelinating lesions not yet visible to the naked eye. The slight changes they detected could therefore reflect the beginning or precursor of the demyelinating process, rather than any preexisting abnormality of the brain tissue wherein demyelination would subsequently take place.[109, 98]

Other studies find that multiple sclerotic blood cells are deficient in linoleate acid. The degree of reduction in the linoleate level appears to correlate with the activity of the disease process. On the other hand, there are studies where no significant difference in acid levels has been found. This discrepancy among findings suggests that the changes relate to the progression of the disease, not ones wrought during the initial synthesis of myelin.

Moreover, there is no certainty whatever that the described decrease in EFAs in the serum lipids is specific to multiple sclerosis; it might just as well be a nonspecific reaction to central nervous system disturbances, or indeed to illnesses in general. In one study, the lowest levels of linoleic acids in serum lipids were present in the most severely incapacitated multiple sclerotics as well as in acutely ill persons, suggesting that the levels are reduced in relation to the severity of the illness. Perhaps the changes in EFA metabolism during sickness are a normal response to acute medical stress, the expected *result* of the disease process and not part of its evolution. Furthermore, the lower serum linoleic acid levels persisted after clinical recovery in three cases of tetanus, three of viral meningitis, one of bacteraemia, one of cortical thrombophlebitis and one of encephalitis.[49]

Several experiments with animals have shown that a severe EFA-deficiency leads to changes in whole brain and brain myelin fatty acid patterns[33,32,1,96] (EFA-deficiency as such has never been found in any case of multiple sclerosis). These changes are much less marked in brain tissue than in other tissues. We know nothing of the course of the changes in brain myelin in humans if EFA restriction occurs during the period of rapid myelination.

While it is debatable whether the almost universal switch from breast to bottle detrimentally affects myelin composition, there is one isolated fact that is often missed. The mother puts some linoleic acid from her diet into her milk and the concentration in the baby's blood is about three times as high in the breast-fed as in bottle-fed babies. The real importance of this difference, I think, is that it is used in making cortisone.[13]

The first attempt to relate changes in brain EFA composition to increased susceptibility to experimental allergic encephalomyelitis (EAE) indicated that a diet adequate in PUFA completely protected rats.*[15,16] Severe flaws in this study prompted other investigators to reexamine the resistance to EAE induced by PUFA-adequate diets, as well as the effects of EFA-deficiency on the developing brain and spinal cord.[82]

The diet of the pregnant rat mother and, subsequently, of her pups had little effect on the lipid constitution of spinal cord myelin, although EFA-deficiency did lead to slightly slower maturation. At early ages the brain also showed signs of slower maturation, but by sixty-eight days of age, there were few differences. And only minor changes were found in lipids in the whole brain and myelin samples.

Nevertheless, EFA-deficiency during central nervous system

---

*EAE, an inflammatory disease of the central nervous system, is generally regarded as an animal model of multiple sclerosis. The term PUFA includes many fatty acids which do not fulfill the requirements for definition as essential fatty acids (EFAs).

development did result in increased susceptibility to EAE. Moreover, a daily oral supplement of the single EFA, linoleic, had a marked protective effect. Clearly, a lack of dietary EFA during development leads to a high susceptibility in the rat to the immunologic insult of EAE. But — and this is critical — the investigators do not feel that there is yet any justification for the view that changes in the myelin membrane lipid composition are the underlying cause of this increased susceptibility. "It has been established that the perivascular infiltrations, which occur during EAE, result from increased vascular permeability, *which indicates an alteration in the protective properties of the BBB*"[82] (italics added). In short, a deficiency of EFAs in the diet during development may render the adult more susceptible to neurologic insult, not as a result of a primary abnormality in chemical composition (lipid or protein) of the myelin sheath, but because of the adverse effect on the BBB.

Classical views on the BBB usually include the notion that it is not present in early life, but develops gradually as the individual develops, to become fully functional only in maturity.

The human brain, among others, undergoes a period of maximum growth that seems to correspond to the second half of foetal life and the first eighteen postnatal months. During this growth spurt the rate of entry of many substances must be greater than at any other time, in accordance with the much greater activity of many metabolic processes. John Dobbing equates this "metabolic performance" of the brain with the BBB. "Until you can show that there is a physical structure interposed between the blood and the brain which limits the rate of a metabolic process by limiting its rate of access to the brain, one has no right, in neurochemical terms, to speak of a blood-brain barrier,"[21] he insists. Instead, he suggests blood-brain relationship (BBR), because it implies function rather than obstruction for a given substance. The BBB for metabolic substances, Dobbing says, can in every instance, be accounted for on the basis of known metabolic behavior. Be that as it may, there is a membrane barrier. The capillaries entering the brain are foreign structures and the brain maintains its basement membrane around every capillary.

The brain growth spurt is regarded as a period of vulnerability, although there are no true deformities, nor any focal tissue destruction. However, numerous data do indicate that permanent metabolic changes are induced by malnutrition in rats during this period. It seems probable though, that a deficit in protein, the backbone of lipid incorporation in the brain and perhaps responsible for the highly complicated lipid substructure, would have a longer lasting deleterious effect on the brain than a transient deficit in EFAs.

What, then are the long-term effects of early damage to the BBR? On the one hand, there is an induced metabolic abnormality that may only be revealed later, if at all, under the modifying effects of some environmental agent(s). On the other, there is an adaptation to a previous environment which persists. This, in effect, is a kind of brain homeostasis which is not a question of permeability at all, but of the control by the brain of its own composition. A predisposition to multiple sclerosis is likely to be largely due to one or the other, rather than to the constitution of the myelin sheath.

The cause of multiple sclerosis is not known, therefore there is no accepted drug therapy. Neither is it a disease that is generally characterised by pain. However, in cases where there is spinothalamic tract involvement, intractable pain is often experienced. To date, two drugs have proved successful in partially alleviating pain in multiple sclerosis, and these may provide some clues regarding etiology.

Once the stage of exhaustion in the battle of adaptation to a particular substance has been reached, avoidance is the only remedy known so far. Substances that can aid resistance or block the allergy, when it affects the brain, have yet to be fully evaluated. Largactil®, which appears to offer some relief of pain, is chemically derived from an antihistamine.

Other drugs that reverse or block allergic reactions, rather than merely reduce the symptoms, are beginning to appear. Dr. Len McEwen of the Wright-Fleming Institute, the leading allergy unit in Britain, has developed a vaccine effective against allergies to many foods. He has incorporated bacteria as well as tiny doses of about fifty common foods in his vaccine. Some of his successes with cases of asthma and hayfever resistant to the conventional pollen-, mould-, and dust-based injections may be due to his taking bacteria into account in the development of food allergy.

The action of Tegretol® in controlling lower back and limb pain in multiple sclerosis, which it does in some cases, is not clearly understood. However, since it is known to control pain in *tic doloureaux*, which can be allergic in origin, it too may act to block the allergic response.[44]

Whether this reasoning is correct or not, whenever an individual presents a history of active ecologic disease, then all other symptoms, however bizarre, must be considered to be related to the underlying allergic predisposition, until proven otherwise. The majority of human allergic responses fortunately conform to a pattern of benign functional reversible states; however, these reactions *can* be more severe and prolonged, resulting in irreversible organic changes. They can occur as acute overwhelming necrotic reactions or, more frequently, by a mechanism of repeated insults to the target organ, due to an unrecognised allergenic etiologic agent.

A chronic ecologic disorder like multiple sclerosis is a multifaceted individual-specific disease. A particular environmental agent may elicit similar or totally different reactions among a group of susceptible individuals with each responding in her own characteristic manner by having an exacerbation of her unique syndrome. The task is to identify and remove the allergenic substance, or if that is impossible, to strengthen the sufferer's powers of adaptation to it. In short, to recognise and *to take into account,* Albert Rowe's statement that allergy, next to infection, is probably the most common cause of human symptomatology.

. . . now . . .

> The present is the going to meet myself as I throw
> myself as what I have become into the future.
>
> J. H. van den Berg[108]

THE certainty of incurable disease emphasizes the blessings of health. It seems that a life of incurable disease is one that cannot be really lived; it must simply be passively endured. Its recognition is an experience of complete surprise, so that one suddenly becomes uncertain about things taken most for granted. It marks the beginning of a long process of inner reconstruction which leads gradually to the realisation that all that has changed is the direction of life, and that is good. My life has a new purpose which it is still within my power to bring into full being.

Being multiple sclerotic, the future appears at first as a muddle of approaching failures. I start each day, fearful and reluctant, and I have good reasons for my apprehension. The stories I have heard about the disease, tragic tales about my inevitable progress from stick to wheelchair to bed, about incontinence and blindness, determine the way I approach tomorrow. They mean that each new day has a terrifying aspect long before it arrives. Unavoidably I greet each one according to the character it has been given by the stories I am told. Is it any wonder that there are more and more days that are so unattractive that I am inclined to turn over again and pretend the day has not begun at all? Being multiple sclerotic, a pitiful future seems very real to me, so real that I have immense difficulty in avoiding being entirely influenced by it now. If I allow myself to be so influenced, any real living can take place only hesitatingly, fearfully. The future is contained in the present, a later apparent to me now, depicted in its starkest terms by the

97

purveyors of doom.

But I refuse to be wholly influenced by a discouraging prognosis. Instead I put my experiences of the past — happy, creative, fulfilling — into the future. In this future, *my* personal future, my past speaks so convincingly to me, beckons me so seductively, that I can do nothing else than embrace it with joy. A glorious past outweighs all fears of the future.

Both past and future have a present value, they are enshrined in the immediate now. The present is a rushing forward beyond myself, a thrusting ahead of what was into what is to come. Being multiple sclerotic, I have chosen a particular form in which to throw my past before me, in which to place myself in the future. It is this that makes it possible, indeed imperative, for me to live on.

The form that I have chosen is caring: not now only to receive care from parents, spouse, friends, but also to give it; no longer just a taker but also a giver. Caring is the centre around which my activities and experiences are integrated. This encourages a harmony between myself and the world that is deep-seated and enduring. It is also my way of thanking for what I have received.

Nonetheless, I cannot care for life in general. I can only thank life by caring for this or that instance of it. I experience each expression of life — a person, an idea, an ideal — as an extension of myself, but also as independent and with the need to grow. Its development is bound up with my own sense of well-being, and I feel needed by it for that growing.

I hope that the expression I choose will grow through my caring, a hope akin to that accompanying the birth of spring. This hope does not contrast the inadequacy of the present with the adequacy of a hoped-for future; rather it celebrates the plenitude of the present, a present alive with a sense of the possible. Such hope rallies energies and activates powers, implying as it does that there is, or could be, something worthy of commitment.

If my carings are inclusive enough, they are deeply involving and fruitfully order all areas of my life. Inclusive ordering means giving up certain things and activities and therefore includes an element of submission that is able to liberate and affirm at a fundamental level. This is like the liberation that comes with the full acceptance of a medically incurable disease: there is acquiescence rather than resignation with lingering resentment, and the realisation with time that it could not be otherwise. Submission entails abandoning pretensions, ceasing to play games, coming to accept myself exactly as I am. I see the conditions of my life just as they are, and not as I might wish them to be.

We are in-place in the world through having our existence ordered by inclusive caring; in short, through our way of relating to others or another expression of life. This introduces something quite new into our own lives, this time like the change occurring when we take full responsibility for ourselves. Place calls for continuous renewal and reaffirmation because it is our response to the need of something to grow which gives it to us.

SECTION II

Universal Oneness

It is all a rhythm
from the shutting
door, to the window
opening.

The seasons, the sun's
light, the moon,
the oceans, the
growing of things
. . . .

The rhythm which projects
from itself continuity
bending all to its force
from window to door,
from ceiling to floor,
light at the opening,
dark at the closing.

—Robert Creeley, in Panati, C.,
   Supersenses, London, Jonathan Cape,
   1975.

THE TREATMENT OF
MULTIPLE SCLEROSIS

Health is a continuing property, potentially measurable by the individual's ability to rally from insults, whether chemical, physical, infectious, psychological or social.

J. R. Audy[2]

ALLERGIC disturbances, like infectious diseases, are generally interpreted in terms of antigen-antibody relationships within the body. In fact, allopathy requires that a known immunologic mechanism be demonstrated before the condition be designated allergic. Allergy to iophendylate, for example, is denied because of a lack of detectable antibody formation after its administration. This trend emphasizing etiology in terms of mechanisms — basic structural formula, molecular size, blood concentration, mechanical displacement of blood by non-oxygen carrying fluid, cholinesterase inhibition by the contrast media, among others — is aided and abetted by advances in physiology and especially pharmacology or, more accurately, pathopharmacology.

The upshot of these developments is the treatment of both infectious and allergic processes by means of drugs aimed to alleviate symptoms or to alter the bodily mechanisms involved, rather than to identify, minimise or neutralise the effect of specific environmental exposures. For instance, infections are treated with broad spectrum antibiotics, irrespective of their specific etiology. Allergies are treated with antihistamines, vasoconstrictors, steroids and other symptomatic measures, irrespective of their environmental causes.

Although this approach, together with improvements in sanitation and other public health measures, has proved reasonably satisfactory for many infectious diseases, our susceptibility

103

to antibiotics and other drugs is becoming more and more commonplace. Increasingly, clinical iatrogenesis is rearing its ugly head, and at least certain chronic and/or complicated infectious processes seem to be multiplying.

This diagnostic-therapeutic orientation to allergic disturbances, being relatively applicable *en masse*, is economical in the short term. But over a longer span of time it has often been relatively expensive and ineffectual. Not only do such programs tend to perpetuate chronic illnesses, they also favour advancement of the disease process, as well as its complications, including widespread drug sensitivities and other adverse reactions. And equally, if not more important, they promote the continued deterioration of the environment. When the external etiologic agents of chronic illness are neither identified nor controlled on a large scale, they come to be regarded as safe and are allowed to proliferate. This is especially true of synthetically derived drugs, chemical air pollutants and many other facets of the so-called chemical environment to which extreme degrees of individual susceptibility can develop.

Unfortunately, this approach was consolidated before the field of allergy and clinical ecology had been adequately explored. The full range of environmental excitants of symptom response had not been isolated or the more advanced systemic disturbances described. Although the role of airborne particles in the etiology of localised manifestations was recognised during the first quarter of the present century, foods and the systemic responses of headache, fatigue, myalgia and arthritis were not recognised until the second quarter. The etiologic role of the wide range of simple environmental chemicals and the advanced mental and behavioral syndromes were not appreciated until the third quarter.

Thus, interest in what was first described as allergy has taken two progressively divergent courses. The one dominant at present focuses on immunologic and other analytic procedures. Clinical manifestations are usually treated nonspecifically and largely with drugs. Little serious effort is made to identify, measure, control or neutralise etiologic environmental exposures or to determine the susceptibility of the individual involved. This point of view is called *clinical immunology*.

Medically speaking, we live today in an age of immunology. The thrust of all contemporary medical research, indeed of all medical thought, is immunologic. When we consider that our immune system evolved in defence of life itself, it is startling to realise that its sole concern is, quite simply, surfaces. It responds to these alone, whether they surround live cells or dead; whether bacteria, viruses, fungi or chemicals, countering anything it identifies as not-self, the champion of our identity. Thus is the battle for life fought, surface against surface, as every attempt to graft a piece of skin or transplant an organ vividly illustrates.

Unravelling the mysteries of our immune system has been a slow and painstaking affair. The first glimmer was shed by the discovery that we have within us circulating white cells (granulocytes) which store bacterial inhibitors and poisons. At the turn of the century scientists were aware of two parts to our immune system: a cellular defence comprising the granulocytes (as well as the larger and more sophisticated cells, the macrophages, detected later), and a serum defence of specifically manufactured, though as yet unidentified, blood factors. By the 1810s, experiments with tuberculin — a protein extracted chemically from the cell wall of the bacillus responsible for TB and injected into affected guinea pigs — pointed to a third part: another kind of white cell, the circulating lymphocytes.

Finally, in 1925, Zinsser showed that defence against bacterial or viral invasion was too important for the body to leave to any one system. It therefore made use of several: the cellular system consisting of the granulocytes (which increased in number under bacterial assault) and the lymphocytes (which did likewise on viral invasion), as well as the humoral system made up of a combination of different but very special serum factors. Zinsser proved that in each and every bodily reaction to infection these three parts work together. Which one predominates depends on the kind of infection or type of material injected.

Only in 1937, however, did scientists establish exactly what the serum factors participating in the immune response were. Using electrophoresis, a process that exploits the differing electric charges of proteins, Tiselius found three groups of proteins in human blood, each migrating at its own rate. He called these the gamma globulins: alpha, beta and gamma. Collectively, we know them as antibodies because they are the blood proteins produced in response to bodily attacks by foreign substances, or antigens. Now antibodies could be separated from the nonimmunologic proteins in the blood, concentrated and experimented upon. Eleven years later, in 1948, Fagraeus demonstrated that they are made by special cells in the body's bone marrow and lymph nodes; he called these plasma cells. Afterwards it was found that even these derive from activated lymphocytes. But fourteen years more were to pass before a genuine understanding emerged of what antibodies are, what they are made of and how they work.

Antibodies are really nothing more than special proteins circulating in our bloodstream. Made up of linked amino acids, proteins are structurally solid and stable compounds; as such, they constitute the building blocks of the body. In addition, they are able to couple with the surfaces of certain foreign materials. The antibody protein comprises two identical light and two identical heavy chains of amino acids.

The gamma globulins differ in size, amino acid sequence, as well as in respect of the site in the body where they do their attacking. Immunoglobulin A (IgA) is secreted in our tears and saliva and is present in all our mucous membranes. The other two antibodies circulating in the bloodstream are Immunoglobulin G (IgG) and Immunoglobulin M (IgM), the latter being larger and less mobile than the former.

Despite nature's ingenuity there is a critical weakness in our antibody system. Before manufacture of the appropriate IgG and IgM antibodies can begin, the microbes or poisons must be present within the body. The first antibodies we make are always of the IgM type. Being larger than the others, they are less liable to destruction and the most lethal to invaders. But a day or two after any infection begins our plasma cells suddenly stop producing the more effective IgM antibodies and unexpectedly switch to creating the smaller, less potent IgG type.

Antibodies are manufactured by cells in our body in response to foreign markers, or epitopes, on the surface of attacking microbes or poisons. About ten amino acids may contribute to the pattern of an epitope. The replacement of just one amino acid by another in a chain of protein frequently leads to the display of a different epitope. These epitopes, or molecular configurations, differ from those in the membranes of our body's own cells and in the materials we make for ourselves. The large molecules that display epitopes, that are under genetic control, are called antigens; it is against the antigens on a foreign cell's surface, or an injected toxin, that antibodies are made.

What, in essence, antibodies do is very simple. Once the attacking organism breaches the outer defences and enters the body, the antibodies already made against the invader couple with the antigens on its surface and cling to the cell wall of the bacterium or virus. The antibody fits snugly onto the antigen. If the foreign substance is a poison, the antibody is able to neutralise the antigen, so that the toxin circulates harmlessly.

The situation with microbes is different; the antibodies do no actual harm to the bacteria or viruses, but once attached to the microbes surface, unlock a series of physical events leading to its death. Besides antibodies and white cells our immune system has a group of nine separate proteins made in the liver and delivered to our circulation system in vast amounts. Taken together the nine constitute the complement system; the individual proteins are called, in order, C^1, C^2, C^3, all the way up to the final complement, C^9. The name was based on an early misunderstanding of the function of these proteins. The first immunologists thought they complemented the action of the antibodies. In fact, it was the other way round; the antibodies complement the action of the nine serum proteins.

When an antibody molecule couples with its antigen on a microbe's surface, it somehow changes its shape. This change opens up a special area somewhere on the antibody molecule. This site, now exposed to the circulation, activates any passing C^1, the first component of the complement system. It combines with the active area of the antibody already formed on the surface of the microbe. With that it, too, changes shape. A new combining site opens up in it and C^2, the second protein component of complement passing by in the bloodstream, fixes to that. This activates the third component, and so on until all nine are assembled on the bacterial surface. None can be activated until the component directly preceding it has been, and with the final activation of the ninth complement protein, a hole is blasted through the outer wall of the bacterium — the microbe is literally blown apart. It is all over within tenths of a second, long before the bacterium can divide or even try to move away.

But even this discovery did not complete the picture of our immunologic system. Antibodies, evidently, are not the critical element because infants born with immunodeficiency diseases, that is, without the ability to make immunologic agents, do not die immediately; they may live for a year or two. In the early 1950s, Louis Pillemer began a series of experiments that revealed a nonimmunologic protein made in the liver and circulating in the blood which was not an antibody but could still combine with the surface of microorganisms and activate the complement system. He called it properdin.

Evidently, to bridge the gap between microbial invasion and the production and circulation of the correct antibody, the body developed this nonimmunologic protein. It can attach itself to any bacterium getting through the skin, no matter what the type, activate complement and blast the microbe apart before it can penetrate further into the body, and well in advance of any antibody reaching it.

Our bodies are protected by an immunologic system of diverse and complicated parts. As such, it obviously needs some central coordinator. How else could the body know what antibodies to make? Why do some reactions contain granulocytes and others lymphocytes? What directs its functions? Where is it?

It was Robert A. Good, a paediatrician with an outstanding mind, who eventually synthesized what was known about immunology. He showed that our entire immune system, except for the granulocytes, is produced by the cells or lymphocytes making up the lymph nodes. These way stations, scattered throughout the body, are connected by very thin-walled channels running alongside our arteries and veins; these comprise the second great, if poorly understood, circulatory system. Everything immunologic that happens in our body stems from the white cells with no granules, filling every lymph node and travelling so persistently back and forth. Even twenty years ago lymphocytes were not thought to have anything to do with the immune system, something that seems incredible now that they are known to constitute it!

All the lymphocytes that circulate in the tissues have arisen from precursor cells in the bone marrow. About half of these lymphocytes, the T-cells, have passed through the thymus gland on their way to the tissues; the other half, the B-cells, have not. These cells look identical under the microscope, but behave quite differently when coming to our defence. The outer parts of each lymph node is filled with B-cell lymphocytes, the inner parts with T-cells. Every so often a few are released into the bloodstream to circulate throughout the body. These messenger lymphocytes are able, somehow, to detect an antigen (a foreigner) pick it off, carry it back to the nearest node, touch the appropriate lymphocytes (either T or B), thereby transferring the information.

This antigen information activates either the humoral (B-cell) or the cellular (T-cell) part of our immune response. Our antibodies, complement, properdin, granulocytes and macrophages protect us against bacteria and fungi. In reacting to an unknown bacterium, one to which antibodies do not yet exist, the messenger lymphocyte goes to the B-cell area of the lymph node. A B-cell immediately begins to change into a plasma cell, virtually a protein factory making antibodies to fit exactly the antigen brought back by the circulating lymphocyte. In its passage through the lymph node, one messenger lymphocyte can touch thousands of separate B-cells, stimulating each to form a plasma cell. Acting together these produce billions of specific antibodies which, released into the bloodstream, will flood the infected areas and deal with the attacking microbes.

Our other enemies, viruses and parasites, must be handled differently. Viruses are intracellular microbes. They infect us by getting inside our cells, taking over the cell's own protein machinery, making the cell produce more of them instead of the protein or compounds it usually makes. Eventually, the virus kills the cell and then moves on to infect its neighbours. Antibodies can be made against some viruses to prevent them from getting into the cells in the first place. But the majority of viruses infect us by travelling internally from cell to cell; they never expose themselves to our humoral defences. Our cellular defences evolved against these intracellular enemies.

During viral infections a messenger lymphocyte will eventually come into contact with a viral-infected cell. Such a cell is so sick that even its surface structure is changed; the configuration of proteins making up its outer membrane becomes slightly different. The circulating lymphocyte picks up this antigen and returns to the T-cell area of the nearest lymph node. Touching a T-cell causes it to transform itself into an incipient killer lymphocyte. This seeks out a virally infected cell and couples with the antigen on its surface, thereby triggering its internal protein-killing machinery. Coupling with the infected cell is the chemical switch that transmutes the T-cell into a killer cell. Chemical compounds form within the lymphocyte. These pass from it into the infected cell, kill the virus, stop the viral spread and thus give our body the chance to regenerate itself.

Recently, subpopulations of T-cells have been identified. Called regulator cells, they comprise the effector or killer cells that directly attack foreign substances; helper cells that assist other kinds of immune system cells; suppressor cells that "turn off" overreactions to specific antigens; and nonspecific suppressor cells that turn off reactions to almost everything. These last react indiscriminately and so, theoretically, could put the body out of action altogether. We do not know how suppressor cells exert their inhibitory influence over the immune system; it might be through direct contact or via a soluble substance they release. It is suspected, however, that while most of the lymphocyte population in humans decrease with age, suppressor cell activity does not; in fact, it seems to increase — rather a nasty thought.

By 1965 it was obvious that our immune system is one reason for our survival as a species. Who could doubt that our antibodies, our granulocytes and macrophages, our complement and properdin, were responsible for our bodily protection and continued existence? But often the same mechanism for defence can be complicating and hazardous because the reaction which is set up starts off a chain called hypersensitivity reactions. A baby fed on cow's milk that is full of foreign proteins may develop just such a reaction. The infant produces a reactive protein(s) which reacts back with the foreign substance specifically. An infant may carry in his serum a very high titre of antibodies against the proteins in cow's milk. If so, the infant is allergic; he has an altered reactivity to milk which he did not have before getting these antibodies. The degree of hypersensitivity reaction can be very serious. In a few babies it is fatal, leading to the little understood tragedy called sudden unexpected death (SUD), usually around three months of age.

Another kind of complication is seen in the strange disease that often followed injection — prior to the discovery of antibiotics — of horse serum containing antibodies against human disease-causing bacteria. Some of those who received a second shot, even if they recovered from their infection, developed fever and joint pains within a fortnight; a few showed blood and protein in their urine; some even had skin rashes. A third injection could kill the person, and a number did die from the disease that was named, appropriately, serum sickness.

Long after the serum injections ceased, investigations on rabbits continued in an effort to find the cause of the puzzling disease associated with them. Eventually, the blood to be injected was fractioned into its components: sugars, fats, carbohydrates and proteins. Injecting each pure fraction revealed that the disease only occurred after the second injection of protein. The first provoked the production of antibodies by the rabbit's immune system. Their blood was removed and examined and a marked increase in circulating antibodies specific for serum protein found. Within hours after the second injection there was a gigantic increase in antibody levels and with it, the beginnings of disease. A terrifying bodily reaction followed a third injection: almost instantaneously the animals' lungs filled with fluid, their inflamed vessels burst open and bled, their hearts dilated, their kidneys turned white, and minutes later the animals were dead.

Not every rabbit injected with the protein was affected in this way. Hundreds were used, all receiving the same quantity, yet not all developed serum sickness. The mystery was compounded by the fact that the survivors were those whose immune systems, for some odd reason, did not produce vast amounts of antibody against the injected material. The conclusion forced on the incredulous investigators was that the disease was caused by the rabbits' own antibodies produced against the proteins which were mistakenly read as foreign. If the circulating antigen-antibody complexes got stuck in the kidneys, the rabbit acquired kidney disease; if they were deposited in the joints, there was joint disease; in the skin, skin rashes. If they were deposited all over, death quickly ensued.

Serum sickness is the first documented example of an autoimmune disease: that is, one in which the individual's immune system makes antibodies against its own tissues. But what caused the production of these antibodies? What were they made against? Again, a kind of chain reaction occurred: antibodies were made by the recipient against the "foreign" cells of the injected substance. However, their surfaces, although somewhat changed, were still so similar in structure to the surfaces of the recipient's own normal cells that the antibodies produced to counter the invader cross-reacted with them; in short, the antibodies attacked the foreign cells as well as the normal cellular constituents of the recipient's body, thereby causing disease. Clearly, we are capable of making antibodies or, more accurately, autoantibodies against ourselves. Powerful as our immune system is in protecting us, it can be just as relentless in pursuing our destruction.*

---

*This reinforces the view emerging from Selye's work that *defensive operations* are the key to an understanding of disease. David Bakan has extended the argument to the psychological realm.[4] He points out that Selye's conclusions are congruent with Freud's hypothesis that all living substance is bound to die from internal causes.[29]

Not only does our immune system protect us from outside invaders; it also mounts guard against those inside us as well. It is a system which performs the dual function of surveillance and destruction. Our body, we know, is always replacing itself; for every cell that is lost or worn out, a new one exactly like it takes its place. Simple mechanical errors of replication, or mutations, are bound to occur, probably more often than we realise. But our immune system recognises and destroys them before they can grow and divide. This internal control is as crucial to our survival as our ability to fend off outside attackers.

Sometimes, though, the functions of the immune system apparently can be hideously deranged and the two most dreaded modern diseases, multiple sclerosis and at least some of the cancers, are regarded by many as exemplifying aberrations of our life-preserving force. On the one hand, multiple sclerosis is commonly regarded as an autoimmune disease or, more properly, as one with an immunologic basis in which lymphocytes, for one reason or another, have become sensitised to brain and mount an attack on that organ. On the other hand, some cancers may represent a slackening or failure in surveillance that permits abnormal cells to grow and divide, gradually coming to dominate the organ in which they arose. Cancers generally occur in the very young and the old, two groups in which the immune system is not properly functional, either because it is not fully developed or because it has begun to wear out. However, it is likely that something more than a defective immune response is involved in both multiple sclerosis and cancer — the genetic constitution of the individual.

"Freud allowed the death instinct to be served by the self-preservative instincts . . . [He] wrote that 'the instincts of self-preservation of self-assertion and of mastery . . . are component instincts whose function it is to assure that the organism shall follow its own path to death, and to ward off any possible ways of returning to inorganic existence other than those which are immanent in the organism itself.'" Bakan then suggests that the way in which events take place *automatically* in the individual is what Freud identified as reflecting the work of the death instinct. This latter, Selye's diseases of adaptation, as well as autoimmune diseases, "may be identified with those automatic mechanisms in the organism, the primitive, elementary and instinctual mechanisms, which are phenomenologically extraneous to the conscious ego." (See also Appendix I.)

Strange antibodies have been found in the serum of multiple sclerotics, autoantibodies that seem to be made against parts of the multiple sclerotic's own brain. Why are these antibodies produced? What, after approximately twenty years of life, causes the multiple sclerotics' own brain tissue suddenly to be read as foreign and attacked by her own immune system?

Antigenic abnormality in multiple sclerosis may develop over time in different ways. This is true of some cancers where industrial exposures have produced a slowly developed pathology. For example, 100 percent of the workers in a plant distilling β-naphthylamine develop cancer of the bladder. Mesothelioma, a rare cancer which attacks the chest and stomach walls, is now appearing in individuals exposed to airborne asbestos particles. The gestation period in both cases is twenty years or more. During this period each day of exposure produced some small increment of change, the sum of which was finally manifest in gross pathology.[105]

Whatever the etiology of multiple sclerosis proves to be, it is probable that immunologic processes play some part in the evolution of the clinical picture. Their possible involvement is usually discussed in terms of two major concepts: immune deviation and autoimmunity. The former characterises a failure of the immune system to react to certain antigens, combined with a normal or often excessive production of antibody. This condition is common to another disease of the central nervous system (subacute sclerosing panencephalitis), where a chronic measles virus infection is combined with an inadequate immune response to measles antigen and high titres of antimeasles antibodies.

There is evidence that in multiple sclerosis something similar occurs. Various measles antibodies produced locally within the brain have been found in the cerebrospinal fluid as well as specific antibodies against certain components of measles virus. Since there are no reported cases of recurring measles — one attack supposedly gives life-long immunity — the virus must lie dormant in the brain from the time of the original attack. The initial immune failure permitting the virus to escape could be due to altered PUFA membrane concentrations which affect the lymphocyte response to the measles virus. The envelope of the virus represents a modified segment of the cell surface membrane, and on infection fuses with it. Changes in membrane composition might lead to alteration or masking of the antigenicity of the virus or to modification of the cell-virus interaction.

The body's immune system obviously destroys most of the originally invading measles viruses, but some, getting into a few of the blood cells, are able, for reasons unknown, to hide there and survive. During this dormant period the body ignores them, or else after the initial childhood attack the hidden viruses are so adequately shielded from the body's defences that the immune system is never able to reach them.

When they begin to grow in the cells where they have been harboured for so long, perhaps in the wake of stress, the body's immune system responds. In an effort to destroy the growing viruses (or at least to isolate them and prevent them from infecting other brain cells) the infected brain is subjected to a massive immune reaction. This is so powerful that infected cells and normal cells in the immediate area of battle are destroyed together.

In most cases an immune response is life saving. But unlike other tissues, a brain cell once destroyed is destroyed forever: virus or immune reaction, when a brain cell begins to degenerate it is gone and can never be replaced. In the case of a viral brain disease, the body's own defences once brought into play only add to the neuronal destruction being caused by the virus. Recognising this, efforts have been made to restore the appropriate immune response to the measles virus, using the transfer factor, which is a form of immunopotentiation therapy.

On the other hand, primary demyelination may be the result of autoimmune destruction of autologous myelin. There are, in the blood of some multiple sclerotics, lymphocytes that are sensitised to myelin basic protein; in these cases, there is a possibility that an autoimmune type of demyelination is taking place. But it is also possible that the proportion of cells sensitised to myelin basic protein is very low and their contribution to demyelination in multiple sclerosis negligible. An important point is that where demyelination occurs as a result of an autoimmune process, even if the initiating antigen is removed, the autoimmune demyelination is likely to be progressive. Indeed this process may underlie the progressive course of the disease from the very onset seen in a small minority (about 10%) of cases.

An alternative possibility is that myelin is damaged as a nonspecific consequence of a specific cell-mediated immune reaction occurring to an antigen in the vicinity of a myelinated nerve. In this situation it would be possible for a wide variety of different agents to provoke primary demyelination simply as a consequence of cell-mediated immune reactivity in their neighbourhood. In other words, myelin is damaged as a non-specific consequence of a specific delayed-type hypersensitivity reaction directed at a nonnervous tissue antigen.

The mechanism of "bystander" demyelination is not unlike that involved in hay fever. In this bystander-type immune disease the tissues of the allergic person are injured because they are near the destructive chemical reaction of the immune response. In hay fever the antigen is not a foreign circulating protein as it is in serum sickness, but pollen grains. Our immune system goes after these as if they were alive. But since they are not they cannot be killed. They just stay on the surfaces, where the body blindly throws more and more IgA antibodies, more and more complement, more and more lymphocytes at them. The whole area surrounding the pollen grains — the bronchus, the lining of the eyes, the mucous membranes of the nose — becomes the battlefield. The chemical mediators (histamine, serotonin) released by the antibody reaction pulverise the normal tissues (the innocent bystanders) on which the pollen grains sit. They stay where they are while the cells around them are damaged by the chemical mediators, becoming swollen and reddened and keeping us miserable, unable to breathe or to see normally.

Antihistamines do not remove the pollen grains or prevent our antibodies coupling with them. All they do is interfere with the effect of the chemical mediators secondary to the immune reaction. They stop the swelling of the normal tissues, the mucous production, the inflammation and the itching that is the result of the immune response. The pollen grains may still be there, the antibodies still produced, but injury to the surrounding tissues is reduced.

If hay fever is not as deadly an immune complex disease as serum sickness, it is because the immune reactions that occur in the sufferer are restricted to the surface of her body, not to deeper organs. But the skin and the central nervous system have the same origin — ectoderm. It is not unreasonable to assume, therefore, that both are subject to similar reactions to antigens.

Henryk Wiśniewski investigated cell-mediated demyelination in the optic nerve system of the rabbit.[107,108] The rabbit eye, apparently, is an ideal system to explore the immunologic histopathology of the demyelinating process, because there are myelinated nerve fibres within the retina, and the vitreous humour behind is able to retain the test antigens. The pattern of demyelination was studied in animals, some being sensitised by injection to brain specific antigen (central nervous system myelin) and others to indifferent (nonnervous tissue) antigen. After sensitisation, the rabbits were challenged by intravitreous injection of different protein substances. Three days later they were sacrificed and the portion of the optic nerve containing the myelinated fibres examined. All the vessels in this area showed perivascular cuffs of inflammatory cells predominantly of the mononuclear type. The whole rim of nerve fibres below the limiting membrane was infiltrated by these cells and all were demyelinated.

Demyelination took place irrespective of the antigen used, so that whatever was injected into the vitreous to bring in the sensitised cells caused extensive demyelination. Primary demyelination to sensitisation by brain specific antigen, as well as the indifferent type, suggests that the same kind of lesion can be induced by any antigen eliciting a cell-mediated immune response. These findings are important in interpreting the lesions of multiple sclerosis, because similar changes will be observed when cells are "called in" as a result of "immunisation" to brain constituents, or to virus, in fact to *any* other antigen which finds its way to the brain and can induce a delayed type of hypersensitivity reaction.

The mechanism of cell-mediated myelin damage is unclear.

The delayed-type hypersensitivity reactions demonstrated by Wiśniewski lead to a mononuclear cell invasion of adjacent myelinated nerves with consequent primary demyelination. This reaction is not necessarily directed against an endogenous myelin antigen (myelin basic protein); instead its target may be an exogenous antigen, one of environmental origin, introduced into the vicinity of the myelinated fibres. This bystander effect suggests that soluble factors released by activated lymphocytes either attack the myelin directly or through recruitment of accessory cells such as macrophages. This seems to be the most plausible explanation since cells specifically sensitised to myelin, or antimyelin antibodies, are absent during the course of this reaction.

The exposure of lymphocytes (both in humans and experimental animals) to influenza and certain other common viruses may greatly influence their response to antigens. Moreover not only do cells from those exposed to banal viral infections develop unusual reactivity, but they appear to be on edge in the sense that they undergo "spontaneous" transformation *in vitro* to a greater degree than normally.[26,27] Such irritability of the cells may persist for some weeks and may occur in the presence of an influenza epidemic even when the person concerned has not suffered obvious clinical infection. Professor Field also points out that the association of onset or episodes of multiple sclerosis with vaccination or other inoculation procedures might also be related to a nonspecific heightening of lymphocyte reactivity in an already critical situation.

It is clear, however, than any antigen finding its way into the central nervous system or the peripheral nervous system, and then attracting cells, could cause both primary and secondary demyelination. Those antigens that, without great difficulty, can find their way into the central nervous system or the peripheral nervous system are allergens and viruses, and perhaps we need to distinguish between infective multiple sclerosis (which is probably preceded by inflammatory change) and allergic/metabolic multiple sclerosis (which may or may not occur in the absence of inflammatory cells).

If the pathogenesis of multiple sclerosis is indeed immune-mediated our problem is two-fold: the sensitised cell seeking an antigen in the myelin sheath or in its myelinating cell which, somehow, must be denied access to the brain, or disarmed locally; and the specific antigen(s) these cells look for in the brain. Apart from the few instances where lymphocytes are sensitised to myelin basic protein, we have to assume that the cells are attracted into the brain by an antigen not yet identified.

If this antigen is a virus, it is highly unlikely that demyelination in multiple sclerosis is a direct result of its cytopathic affect on myelinated cells, because there are no pathologic changes in the oligodendroglia or myelin before the arrival of a cellular infiltrate, i.e. macrophages. (Myelination occurs in two phases: a phase of oligodendroglial proliferation followed by the manufacture of lipid containing myelin sheaths by the established oligodendroglia or glial cells.) Immunosuppressive therapy at the Clinical Research Centre, Harrow, also seems to indicate that virus-induced oligopathic demyelination is not operative in multiple sclerosis. After intensive immunosuppressive therapy all the multiple sclerotics showed some improvement rather than worsening of the clinical symptoms — the expected outcome in conventional viral infection of the central nervous system. Besides, the life-long nature of multiple sclerosis generally, its long periods of health interspersed with unpredictable exacerbations, is not what would be expected from an acute infectious illness, viral, bacterial or fungal. Also, autopsy examinations of multiple sclerotic brains usually show a kind of tissue destruction different from that caused by any known viral disease.

Thus, if a virus is the source of attraction of the cell it is unlikely to be harmful as long as the host's immune system does not launch an attack on it. What does the harm is not the virus but the adverse effect of a hyperacute reaction between virus and immune system. What causes demyelination, then, is not the invader *per se*, virus or allergen, but the interaction between sensitised cell and antigen. Put another way, demyelination is the result of an allergic reaction that depends on an antigen coupling with the susceptible cell.

But what then can we say about those recalcitrant intruders that do not have antigens on their surface: the vapour phase of cigarette smoke (excluding tars and particulates) or that of petrol fumes, for example? With no surface to be read as foreign, how do these activate the bystander mechanism? Are subtle chemical changes, perhaps no more than an amino acid or two, produced in the membranes of the nervous tissue after a long period of exposure? And what about allergens like chemical poisons (food preservatives and dyes) that, even after a considerable time, may elicit only low antigen changes the immune system cannot detect? Apparently, the tendency to activate the bystander mechanism to any aggravation of susceptible myelin — if this is what multiple sclerosis boils down to — points to something beyond the immunologic system.

After the descriptive term *allergy* was redefined immunologically in 1926, food, drugs and chemical environmental exposures, not being adequately explained within this frame of reference, were not considered allergic. At about that time a series of clinical observations of these factors were initiated which laid the foundation for what came to be known as *clinical ecology*.* This examines man's environment for new evidence of etiologic factors capable of impinging on the health and behavior of specifically susceptible persons and manifesting as illnesses. These factors, or allergic conditions, are not necessarily mediated through known immunologic pathways.

Allergy is not in itself a disease; it is merely evidence of a biologic reaction. In the study of central nervous system allergy, therefore, an hypothesis as to the biologic principle involved may be the most important facet in elucidating many of the conditions that are not well understood at present.

The relevant biologic principle is derived from the Darwinian theory of evolution, or rather that aspect of it concerning the remarkable adaptation in all species to their natural environment. "Evolution in biology," says Julian Huxley, "is a loose and comprehensive term applied to cover any and every change occurring in the constitution of systematic units of

---

*This orientation is based on material contained in the handbook on clinical ecology, edited by Lawrence D. Dickey, M.D.[22]

animals and plants . . .[42] Although there is disagreement over exactly how such changes take place, there is none over the fact that they do. Adaptation, universal in extent and profound in degree, was securely linked by Darwin with time. This is of great importance in biology generally, for we are constructed of bones, flesh — and time. It is time that gives order to the endless activity within the human body.

Time is also of the essence in multiple sclerosis where it is expressed in the periodicity of the attacks. Everyone acknowledges the fluctuations of both signs and symptoms during the course of the disease. Most sufferers report differences in their power and ability during the day and at evening time. Many feel much better at night and may even be able to walk, though they have to use a wheelchair during the day. The same person is one day able to lift up his stretched leg to 60 or 80° and the next to only 30 or 40°. Dr. Torben Fog has shown himself to be particularly sympathetic to, and interested in, these rhythmic changes, as well as the activity within the central nervous system that underlies them, going so far as to say that an acute phase is merely the tip of the iceberg.

The observable reactions of the total living individual to environmental insults can be adequately dealt with in terms of general adaptation as this has been elaborated by Professor Selye. However, the allergic state is one of potential specific reactivity. As such, it is the related clinical concept of specific adaptation, the ability of the individual to adjust to the changing circumstances of her existence, that accounts for the gradations between true-being and false-being; that is, between health and disease.

The techniques of clinical ecology are designed to identify, quantify, eliminate, and/or neutralise specific environmental exposures. In contrast to clinical immunology, specific diagnosis and treatment consist of an interdigitating continuum. Drug therapy is minimised and usually unnecessary. Although the clinical work-up is highly individualised and more time-consuming, and therapy is often restrictive, clinical results tend to be relatively superior in that advancement of the process, and adverse complications are far less apt to occur.

The concept and application of clinical ecology differs from clinical immunology and many other aspects of allopathic medicine in that both the environmental exposure(s) and the vulnerable individual in their constant state of interreaction, are regarded as biologic wholes. It is the dynamic interreaction that is important — the totality of the response arising from the thrusts and parries which characterise this phenomenon in its holistic form as it is encountered in nature. In other words, clinical ecology is not static, the components of which are analysed *ad absurdum*. What the clinical ecologist is interested in is a totality as dynamic and reactive as a pot of bubbling porridge, as Dr. Randolph picturesquely puts it.

Clinical ecologists are not uninterested in the mechanisms of these man-environment interrelationships which are accentuated in the presence of individual susceptibility. Although they are not readily understood at present, they are undoubtedly multiple and include metabolic, endocrine, enzymatic and, of course, many of an immunologic nature.

Multiple sclerosis is an ecologic disease and, as such, falls within the scope of clinical ecology which, in summary, is "concerned with observation and treatment of disease in the individual as distinguished from an artificial experiment in the branch of biology which treats of the relations between organisms and their environment."[22] Put another way, the focus of the clinical ecologist is not an organism in an environment, but a being in an ecosystem.

The diagnostic and therapeutic techniques of the clinical ecologist derive from a working knowledge of the stages of specific adaptation occurring in the presence of individual susceptibility. This provides the means of reverting a chronic illness of obscure origin into an acute illness, thereby demonstrating the inciting and perpetuating ecologic causes of the chronic syndrome. In addition to relieving chronic symptoms, the degree of specific susceptibility and the tendency of this process to spread to related materials can be reduced. Identification and avoidance of incriminated environmental constituents is more rational and effective than merely treating the effects of the illness. Where the disease is too far advanced for this to be successful, other ways must be found to strengthen the individual's powers of adaptation. Ideally, the responses of chronically ill persons to controlled variations in their intake and surroundings are observed in an ecologic unit. At present there are very few of these.

It is well known that multiple sclerosis manifests differently in different people. Its patterns are as idiosyncratic as the etiologic factors that are responsible. Thus, to keep symptom-free may mean such a vast restructuring of home, working conditions and eating habits, that sufferers will undertake it only when they have been seriously ill for a long time and are utterly convinced of the soundness of the ecologic approach.

Paradoxically, the chronically ill person will often reject a new interpretation of her illness which threatens to infringe upon her freedom. Even though she may be intensely interested in learning the causes of her symptoms she is usually loath to accept the restrictions and changes that are demanded. For one thing, although the suggestion that multiple sclerosis results from daily exposures to which one is susceptible may sound reasonable to the thinking person, the brain-fagged, confused or depressed are likely to react negatively to it. In the long run, however, they are more amenable than the euphoric person who does poorly in *any* rehabilitative setting, apparently seeing no reason to strive to fulfill her program. Others are too tired to be attentive; too dull to grasp what is being said; too embarrassed to ask questions and, above all, too habituated in their daily routines and too lacking in initiative to make any substantial alterations. These difficulties are compounded by the advance of the illness. Preoccupied with their own one-track recurring thoughts, the victims cannot comprehend, decide or accept responsibility for themselves. It is far easier to drift into a downward spiral than to make far-reaching changes, even though such upsets might demonstrate the etiology of their own unique syndrome.

It was my considerable good fortune that I was so ill as a result of the pollution of my body by synthetic chemicals that I simply had no option but to discard my life-style. Disease is often nature's way of issuing a warning, and the answer is not so much to overcome the disease as to recognise what nature is trying to say. The relevant insights were not instantaneous, there was no overnight revolution, nothing came easily, and the task is still far from complete. But today, as symptom-free as I will ever be, I believe whole-heartedly that it was worth every ounce of the effort. I believe that success in the fight against multiple sclerosis, exacerbated or not by clinical iatrogenesis, is within the grasp of the majority of sufferers: provided they make the necessary sacrifices and adaptations; provided they are prepared to resist and overcome cultural iatrogenesis; and provided they do not again fall prey to those deeply ingrained habits and daily practices (often unconscious) that made them vulnerable to the disease in the first place.

MULTIPLE SCLEROSIS IS A
PERSONAL AFFAIR

MULTIPLE sclerosis is a degenerative, chronic disease which affects the central nervous system. Its early diagnosis, in itself a crucial event in the adaptation process, depends mainly on three individuals: first, the sufferer. The danger signals are many and unpredictable; each symptom, by itself, could herald one of a number of disorders. But a combination of three or more simultaneously, or in succession, could be a warning of multiple sclerosis. Never ignore these; see your general practitioner at once. It may very well *not* be multiple sclerosis. But let your doctor tell you. Don't guess. The danger signals that could mean multiple sclerosis include:

Partial or complete paralysis of parts of the body
Numbness in parts of the body
Double or otherwise defective vision, such as involuntary movements of the eyeballs
Noticeable dragging of one or both feet
Severe bladder or bowel trouble (loss of control)
Speech difficulties, such as slurring
Staggering or loss of balance
Extreme weakness or fatigue
Pricking sensation in parts of the body
Loss of coordination
Tremor of hands

Of special significance is the unexplained disappearance of one or more of these symptoms, either permanently or temporarily. They may vanish for several years at a time and, occasionally, never return. In general, whatever the individual was doing while getting better receives the credit for this kind of remission, but no one knows, as yet, why this occurs in some people, while in others the disease progresses steadily. The general practitioner, the second link in the diagnostic chain, is usually not consulted until one or more relapses have occurred.

When someone has one of the above symptoms and the clinical examination is negative, its disappearance may reassure both her and her doctor. The emphasis in medical training on the diagnostic importance of signs rather than symptoms could allay any suspicion of early multiple sclerosis.

The final link is the consultant, usually a neurologist, who diagnoses. It is well known how very difficult it can be to diagnose multiple sclerosis. The early symptoms and signs are vague and can mimic any disease of the brain and spinal cord. Very often the findings of a clinical examination are negative. If conditions that simulate multiple sclerosis, notably tumour of the brain or spinal cord are suspected, some tests may be necessary. These are undertaken reluctantly because "myelograms or pneumoencephalograms (air encephalographs) can themselves be sufficiently traumatic to exacerbate multiple sclerosis. A complicating factor is that the demyelination process can itself produce a positive brain scan that simulates a tumour."[13]

In the end, diagnosis depends on the clinical judgment of the neurologist and since this is notoriously unreliable, make sure that the consultant has exercised it in respect of this disease on many occasions in the past. Experience of the disease is essential, but many neurologists, particularly in the Southern Hemisphere where multiple sclerosis was very rare until recently, are relatively unfamiliar with it. They also tend to prevaricate, calling it a demyelinating disease, polyneuritis, cerebellar ataxia, almost anything but multiple sclerosis. Nothing could be more true than the truthful lie and yet communicate less truth to the person. Some neurologists, apparently, leave the room as soon as they have delivered their judgment and will discuss the disease only when pressed hard to do so. As more than one sufferer has told me: multiple sclerotics are treated like dirt.* In fairness, however, perhaps the only way that a

---

*My own case was so bizarre that I felt compelled to record it in detail in *The Medical Cop-Out* (Cape Town: Human & Rousseau, 1976.)

doctor can be reasonably certain of a diagnosis of multiple sclerosis is to follow the individual's progress for some years.

In a clinical examination the *optic discs* are studied by means of an ophthalmoscope. There may be pallor on the temporal side of the disc with occasional slight swelling. However, they are usually normal in appearance during an acute attack unless the eyes are directly affected.

Pain behind the eyes due to *retrobulbar neuritis* (inflammation of nerves behind the eye) can be acute, and any movement of the eyeball causes severe distress. Permanent blindness is rare, although transient central scotoma (a blind area in the field of vision) is not uncommon.

The *pupils* are tested for reaction to light by using a torch, which causes constriction when the light is on and dilation when the light is removed. Accommodation is tested by moving an object (such as a pencil) from a distance of about a foot away gradually towards the eyes.

Muscle reactions are tested by striking the muscle tendon with a small rubber hammer, whereupon the muscles show some response. The knee jerk is obvious when the area just below the kneecap is struck, and the lower leg shoots up. The reaction is exaggerated in some cases and absent in others. A Babinski reflex may be present. The sole of the foot is stroked — usually with the blunt end of the reflex hammer in a manner that leaves an indelible impression on the skin, and in the mind that all neurologists are born sadists — and the big toe bends upwards instead of downwards. Abdominal reflexes are often absent. This is demonstrated by stroking the abdomen from the centre and outwards on both sides, above and below the navel.

Skin sensation is tested by using a pin or cotton wool. In some cases sensation is absent in patchy areas and in others, exaggerated to the extent of generating excessive pain.

X-rays of the skull are taken to exclude any alternative pathology such as a brain tumour. A *lumbar puncture*, withdrawal of cerebrospinal fluid by passing a hollow needle painlessly into the spinal canal, is performed as it is sometimes of value in diagnosis.

No medication has yet been successful in treating multiple sclerosis. Virtually hundreds of drugs have been tried in an effort to influence the course of the disease, but neither these nor other forms of therapy have proved to be consistently beneficial. Although there is no specific treatment, the multiple sclerotic can and should be treated.

Keep in close contact with your general practitioner. Do not ignore his advice now that multiple sclerosis has been named as the source of your troubles. Once you begin thinking that every ache and pain is related to multiple sclerosis you greatly increase your chances of ignoring a problem that may have nothing to do with it. Even if you are multiple sclerotic you can develop other medical problems, both big and little. Pneumonia, broken bones, kidney infections, indigestion, diabetes, high blood pressure are all problems with which your general practitioner becomes involved. He is the one best equipped to pinpoint nonmultiple sclerotic related health hazards, thus saving you a great deal of unnecessary worry.

An infection anywhere in the body can make a person feel weak and less able to cope with any disability. Good general medical care devoted to the prevention of upper respiratory and bladder infections is most important, but even minor infections should be treated without delay. *Do not try to dose yourself by filling your system with patent medicines,* especially those passed on by well-meaning friends or relatives because they have taken them for a similar complaint. A drug that benefits one person may mean death to another. Establishing appropriate patterns of care, including regular visits to the dentist, as soon as possible is merely good sense.

Although there is no cure as such for multiple sclerosis, remission is a distinct possibility in 90 percent of cases, but it is an achievement that does depend to a large extent on the amount of support and help the patient can get from others — family, friends, employers and general practitioners. Furthermore, it is also possible to remain symptom-free, but this state is the full responsibility of the individual herself.

In remission, we must discover, or invent, and exploit any approach that is capable of improving our bodily control of the allergic responses which are the true cause of the multiple sclerotic plaque. Those whose condition is long standing and in whom oft-repeated allergic reactions have caused irreversible physical changes in the tissue, or deeply implanted mental conditioning, can also be helped. But in them the improvement will be only partial, for after many years, pathologic changes of a more permanent nature will usually have taken place. Relapse into an acute phase suggests an addictive element in food, chemical and other allergy.

Since some stress is clearly unavoidable, our object is not to try to eliminate it altogether, but to learn to live with it and minimise its harmful effects. In fact, a certain amount of stress is beneficial. It has been recognised since early times that there is a force in nature, the *vis medicatrix naturae*, which tends to heal from within — keeping the body whole and stable in the face of its enormous potential instability — and that this force is activated by stress.

From the ecologic point of view, then, it is essential that those who develop multiple sclerosis understand, very clearly, that the rate of progress of their disease depends on the pattern of life they plan for themselves.

In the first place, purely psychologic factors are vitally important in that they are capable of raising our powers of adaptation to stresses of all kinds, of which sensitivity to specific foods and chemicals is but one. Multiple sclerosis occurs more frequently in members of the upper social classes in whom the social demands, the weight of responsibilities and of authority, as well as the rat-race type of living, may lead to particular varieties of stress and fatigue.

Moreover, the stressful and fatiguing situations that appear to be dangerous for the MS-vulnerable, seem to differ both as regards age and sex. Thus in respect of the youngest group, girls apparently enter the danger category earlier than do boys. Those who start multiple sclerosis before the age of twenty years are usually girls. They throw themselves at life in a way that is well designed to damage their health, their brains, and especially their blood-brain barriers. On the other hand, at this early age boys are less involved in the battle to "succeed." Their turn comes later, for it is toward the end of their twenties that the struggle for status in a business or profession seems to allow a liability for multiple sclerosis to be realised.

Self-Healing: I

> No one else can give me the meaning of my life; it is something I alone can make. The meaning is not something predetermined which simply unfolds; I help both to create it and to discover it, and this is a continuing process, not a once-and-for-all.
>
> —Milton Mayeroff[51]

The language of diagnosis and treatment of someone said to have multiple sclerosis masks the web of ecologic connections that is the real truth of the matter. An unsatisfied need, an unassuageable gap, can be found in the situation of every multiple sclerotic. Such a gap may be of any type: a chemical or organic hiatus; a wound in emotional being; an isolation approaching limbo in relation to the world. One way or another, there is a gulf which cannot be filled and stay filled.

Of course, we try to fill these holes in a variety of ways. I think most of us look to the technology of medicine in this regard. Lewis Thomas distinguishes here between three quite different levels so unlike each other as to seem altogether different enterprises.[102] First, there is a vast "non-technology," impossible to assess in terms of its capacity to alter either the natural course of disease or its eventual outcome. This is the supportive therapy that helps the sick through diseases that are not understood. It is what is meant by "caring for" and "standing by," and it is indispensable. Doctors used to be engaged in nothing else at the sickbed of people with diphtheria, meningitis, poliomyelitis and all the rest of the infectious diseases that have since come under control. It is what doctors must now do for those with intractable cancer, severe rheumatoid arthritis and multiple sclerosis.

Supportive medical care is not a technology in any real sense, since it does not involve measures directed at the underlying mechanism of the disease. Nevertheless its cost is very high and getting higher all the time. It calls for a great deal of time, concerted effort and skill on the part of the doctor; only the very best are good at coping with this kind of defeat.

At the next level up is a technology Lewis calls "halfway." This refers to things that must be done after the fact, in efforts to compensate for the incapacitating effects of certain diseases whose course we are unable to do much about. It is designed to make up for disease, or to postpone death. The outstanding examples in recent years are the transplantations of hearts, kidneys, livers and other organs; inevitably I suppose, we have arrived at halfway measures for multiple sclerosis.

Paraphrasing from *Medicines in the 1990s:* Fundamental advances in neurologic disorders will have to wait upon the twenty-first century. One forecast suggests that the use of very fine metallic filaments as prosthetic replacements for nerves and nerve channels in the spinal cord may be possible by the year 2020.

To the public, this kind of technology seems to be the equivalent of the high technologies of the physical sciences. The media present each new procedure as a breakthrough and therapeutic triumph, instead of the grotesque makeshift that it really is.

This level of technology is at once highly sophisticated and profoundly primitive. It is the kind of thing we must do until there is a genuine understanding of the interrelationships involved in disease. In multiple sclerosis we need to know more about the formation of myelin before we can intervene intelligently to stimulate the regeneration of whatever has been destroyed. And when this level of understanding is reached, the technology of nerve replacement will not have much place.

The third type of technology is so effective that it attracts the least public notice; it is simply taken for granted. This is the decisive technology of modern medicine that is the result of a true understanding of the disease in question, and when it becomes available, it is relatively inexpensive and easy to deliver. Included are antibiotics for the treatment of pneumonia, tuberculosis and syphilis, hormones for the correction of endocrine functions, nutritional therapy to prevent the manifestation of certain inherited and acquired disorders, and immunisations.

The basic idea of immunisation is to let the body do it, to help the body do it, and to use the body's own massive resources to cure and heal itself. In short, immunisations exploit the body's immunologic defenses, although the early pioneers (among them Pasteur and Jenner) were hardly aware of this. To use the body in this way, to artificially force it to protect itself, has been the greatest achievement of medicine. Yet as Dr. Ronald Glasser aptly remarks, it is an achievement of negatives; its success is related to things that never happen.[35] And in this dramatic age of cardiac pacemakers, open-heart surgery, corneal repairs and kidney transplants, it is difficult to get the public excited or concerned about something that does not happen, or epidemics that occurred 200 years ago, or even fifteen.

Most people would argue that the only thing that can nudge multiple sclerosis toward the arena of high technology is new information, and the only imaginable source of this is basic research. They might compare the halfway technology of the disease with that evolving for polio in the early 1950s, just before the emergence of the basic research that made the vaccine possible. Do you remember Sister Kenny, and the cost of those institutes for rehabilitation, with all those ceremonially applied hot fomentations, and the debates about whether the affected limbs should be totally immobilised or kept in passive motion as frequently as possible, and the masses of statistically tormented data mobilised to support one view over another?

It is when doctors are bogged down by their incomplete technologies, by the innumerable things they are obliged to do because they lack a clear understanding of the disease, that the deficiencies and the grave dangers of the science of medicine are most conspicuous. Basic research, which generally has no immediate application, begins to percolate through into the clinician's outstretched hands. Shortly afterwards the creepy realisation grows that clinical research, no matter how seductive the guise, is the new tyranny of medicine. Drugs are tried, investigations pursued, surgery performed, even though the doctor knows that the real answer may lie in a change of diet or better nutrition.

In reviewing recent experimental developments in multiple sclerosis, Dr. Kelly applauds the encouragement these offer to sufferers as evidence of the intensive efforts that are being made to find a way of treating their disease. But, he continues, we should not be encouraged to believe that if we are not being treated with these experimental methods we are losing out. Instead, there is a considerable possibility that events will show that those who have offered themselves for trials with these methods of treatment have lost out as a result.[44]

Dr. L. A. Liversedge, of the Department of Neurology at the University of Manchester, is equally realistic in his observations on our ideas about a "cure" for multiple sclerosis. "Unfortunately the curative essays in management of multiple sclerosis have been confused by the mysteries surrounding not only the scientific but also the *social, personal and emotional elements* compounding this disorder."[48] The fact is that beyond a certain point no chemical or other therapeutic agent can compensate, indemnify or cover up the needs of the multiple sclerotic because, at root, degenerative disease is a disorder of ecologic organisation. One cannot offer clinical prostheses for broken relationships.

Our health and our diseases can only be understood with reference to *us*, as expressions of our nature, our living. Given certain conditions, we create our own sickness; we imagine and construct innumerable diseases, whole worlds of morbidity that we can defend or destroy. And just as we allow diseases, so we collude with them, and connive at them, greedily embracing sickness and suffering, plotting our own ruin.

But, by the same token, we can resist and combat our own diseases, using not only the remedies which doctors and others provide, but resources and strengths of our own which are inborn or acquired. We would never survive without these powers of health which are, finally, the deepest and strongest we have.

The most powerful resources in degenerative disease are resilience of *attitude* and the infinitude of the human *imagination*. Every multiple sclerotic has a human nature and is subject to all of the vulnerabilities of the human condition. Nothing I have done, or have not done, can alter the fact that I belong to the family of man. I am therefore prone to illness, suffering and pain. None of us is exempt from misfortune. Being multiple sclerotic I am forced to confront my own humanness. I may not wish to accept it, but at least I cannot turn my back on it. As soon as I recognise that painful fate cannot be changed — it would not be fate if it could — I must accept it. Beyond that, I must transmute it into something meaningful, into an achievement.

Knowledge about illness among health professionals is limited to the common disease conditions: the etiology, signs and symptoms and treatment. Our view of disease and suffering is that these are undesirable states to be cured or alleviated as soon as possible. Our diseases are purely alien and bad, without organic relation to the person who is ill. They are entities that take possession of us, ontologic ghouls, things that can be "caught." Our health and diseases are not seen in relation to our being-here-in-the-world. The odd notion that diseases are not part of ourselves and of the world, but outside nature, demonic, allows us to be exempted from responsibility for our condition, and from striving actively for a coherent organisation in which we and what goes on around and inside us are all essential elements.

With the passage of time medicine may banish some diseases, but it will always find others. As new solutions replace the old ones, new problems replace the ones that have been solved. Medicine by no means diminishes illness. On the contrary, it generates it. The professions do not produce goods; they provide services to others. The need for these is largely self-generating, but where needs are not immediately evident, they are manufactured. Advertising is the most obvious activity devoted to creating demands which become needs.

Medicine can interfere increasingly in individual lives by altering the definitions and perceptions of health and illness. Medicine continually raises expectations which, when they are not fulfilled, are classed as illness. States of unease are then seen by the public as disease, and for every disease there must be a cure.

But what is a cure? In the case of acute illness, the answer is easy and it is partly the dramatic improvements in this area that have encouraged the idea that more often than not, cure is possible. However, with chronic illness, unless it is of ecologic origin and there is the means of reverting it to an acute state, the answer is obscure. It is meaningless to speak of cure in relation to many of the cardiovascular disorders, diabetes, many of the collagen diseases, many central nervous system disorders, some of the cancers and so on. Moreover, what was acceptable as a cure in long-standing disease a decade ago, is no longer acceptable as such. Expectations rise with scientific advance, so that relief offered to an arthritic in 1920 might be rejected by one today. Medicine continually seeks new remedies, and the members of the public demand them. Doctors are their one and only saviour, and cultural iatrogenesis is the outcome.

Many people assume, implicitly anyway, that a sick person who is unproductive, bedridden, in pain or completely dependent on others is better off dead. When little can be done in terms of a cure, what is the attitude of medical professionals? Multiple sclerotics are particularly qualified to answer this. Specialists (but nurses as well) tend to view any failure to improve as a reflection on their professional competence. Once they know that a person is incurably ill, medically speaking, they withdraw psychologically and physically, conveying an air of helplessness and hopelessness to the sufferer. "There is nothing we can do" or "she would be better off dead" types of attitudes corrode relationships and may well drive a multiple sclerotic to despair. Something can *always* be done for the multiple sclerotic: she can be helped to find meaning in the very situation that everyone else experiences as totally meaningless.

But where illness is viewed as intrinsically bad, both the sufferer and her doctor are likely to place inordinate value on a "cure," thereby severely hindering the discovery of meaning in being multiple sclerotic.

Illness is a natural, common life experience. This is not to say that it is a positive good, or that it is to be preferred to health. It does mean though that like every other life experience it carries the potential for growth, provided that the sick person and her family can find meaning in it. This is just where the deadening effect of cultural iatrogenesis is most apparent; it is what the multiple sclerotic *must* overcome as the first step in freeing her adaptive powers. Sustained by relationships with other human beings most multiple sclerotics *can* cope with or find meaning in their disease, even though they may not have any hope of a cure.

Moreover, the absence of a cure does not exclude the possibility of a healing and therefore, remission. Healing is not principally concerned with the correction and cure of a physical disability. Rather it involves the reintegration of the forces of the individual's life, the recovery of the pattern and organisation that multiple sclerosis has shattered. As a person, a being with the power of self-awareness, the individual under normal circumstances is generally so poorly integrated that she experiences herself as an assembly of many different personalities, each saying me. The degree of integration, of inner coherence and strength, is closely related to the kind of world that exists for the multiple sclerotic. "As above, so below," the Ancients used to say: to the world outside us there corresponds, in some fashion, a world inside us.

Our five senses extended by a great array of apparatus register the visible things of the physical world. But they cannot detect such fundamental invisible powers as life. The recognition of the fact of life has even led people to assert that "there exists in all living things an intrinsic factor — elusive, inestimable and unmeasurable — that activates life." Yet who could see, hear, touch, taste or smell life as such? It has no shape or colour; no specific sound, texture, taste or smell. Nevertheless, as we can know life, we must have a relevant organ of perception, one more inward and different from the senses. This organ is identical with the life inside ourselves, the involuntary self-regulatory processes and feelings of our living body under the control of the autonomic nervous system.

Healing is achieved through understanding, not only the state of being multiple sclerotic, but also the perfection of which that state is a broken symbol. There must be insight too, into how and when the original perfection began to deteriorate into this base reality. All this is uncovered at the level of being; for in the last analysis, the multiple sclerotic's own body and her own psyche must do their healing; must remit according to their own conception of perfection.

The human being, instead of being driven from behind as most contemporary psychology has it, is pulled from ahead by the challenge of finding meaning in life's experiences. This can be found in illness, suffering and pain, and death, as in any other experience. When it is, the multiple sclerotic can use it to achieve adaptation and that which lies beyond: the transcendence of consciousness to reach the level of self-awareness.

This is not easy, of course. Disease and suffering do not have intrinsic meaning. Only the person experiencing the reality of the disease can ascribe value to it. Meanings originate in a human being, not in a situation. It is the individual involved in and living through the state of being multiple sclerotic who imbues it with meaning. Since each one of us is unique, the meaning which we attribute to being multiple sclerotic is also unique.

Meaning exists to the extent that the multiple sclerotic realises that she is still useful, albeit marginally, in regard to certain tasks which can be performed or fulfilled only by herself. To be useful is to feel necessary, and this gives being multiple sclerotic significance. Just as I may be indifferent to myself, use myself as a thing, or be a stranger to myself, so I may care for myself by being responsive to my own needs to grow. I become my own guardian, as it were, and take responsibility for my own life.

Inducing care for oneself means caring for someone or some other expression of life besides. The question, then, is what might the sufferer be willing to live for? What may rekindle and fan the spark of life within her? Which human beings does she care about? Is there a pet she values? Any idea or cause she might be willing to live for? Any unfulfilled dreams, unfinished work? What fragments of beauty once moved her?

When the incurably ill person wants to discuss the problems of life and death, she finds few who will even listen to her, much less provide an opportunity to explore some possible meanings of these perennial life problems. Thus when assistance from others is most needed, the multiple sclerotic often discovers she is most isolated. She has no option but to grapple with the problem alone. Those who cannot cope conclude that what has happened to them is senseless and inexplicable. The real tragedy is that this is not even recognised by those whose responsibility it is to help and comfort.

Self-Healing: II

> To dismiss the most central fact of man's being because it is inner and subjective is to make the hugest subjective falsification possible — one that leaves out the really critical half of man's nature. For without that underlying subjective flux, as experienced in floating imagery, dreams, bodily impulses, formative ideas, projections, and symbols, the world that is open to human experience can be neither described nor rationally understood. When our age learns that lesson, it will have made the first move toward redeeming for human use the mechanized and electrified wasteland that is now being bulldozed, at man's expense and to his permanent loss, for the benefit of the Megamachine.
>
> —Lewis Mumford[58]

The classification of disease in our society mirrors its organisation: high blood pressure is an alibi for mounting stress; degenerative disease an alibi for degenerating sociocultural organisation. Thus multiple sclerosis, the most common degenerative disease of the nervous system, must be approached metaphysically, as pattern and design. Its forms and transformations are infinitely varied; individuality is its principal characteristic. But common to all of its victims is the sense of pressure, coercion and force; the insidious encroachment of pathologic rigidity and insistence.

For the healthy adult, her experience of herself both as a full participant in and as completely separate from the "world-out-there," is simply taken for granted. Consciousness of self and absorption without awareness of self are polarities between which each of us moves with varying degrees of ease. As we develop, personal integrity, which in the early years is entirely physiologic, takes on ethical and psychologic qualities. At these more advanced symbolised dimensions, the individual will disintegrate if her interior models, her inner forms and images becomes deficient representations of her being-in-the-world and, therefore, inadequate bases for thinking and acting.

There is nothing more difficult than to become critically aware of those fundamental assumptions we ordinarily make about our world. A special effort, an effort of self-awareness, is needed. This is a rare power, precious and vulnerable in the extreme, a supreme and generally fleeting achievement, present at one moment and all too easily gone the next. Self-awareness is not merely an intensification of consciousness; it is a separate power having nothing automatic or mechanical about it. It is essentially a limitless potentiality rather than an actuality. It has to be developed and realised by each of us if we are to become persons. And once a human potentiality is realised, it exists.

In the ongoing flux of life we undergo many changes and every change involves both a loss and a gain. Like stress, loss can have many meanings and, like stress, it tends to be a *post hoc* attribution; that is, we do not know until after it has occurred whether being multiple sclerotic can be construed as a loss or a gain. Or the pros and cons may balance out so evenly that it cannot be interpreted as one or the other. But no matter how we see the situation, the crucial factor is the way we adapt to the changes intrinsic to being multiple sclerotic.

We can deal with the clash between the world we once knew and the one we inherit on becoming multiple sclerotic in different ways. One is to abandon totally our former view of the world. We try to put out of mind what we could once achieve and concentrate instead on whatever future remains to us. This is most likely to succeed if we have a relatively realistic conception of our new world, of what it means to be multiple sclerotic, so that we can accept it with equanimity.

However, the consequences of rejecting altogether old models are not always beneficial, either to the person in transition or to others affected by her behavior. During the weeks immediately following the diagnosis, it is easy for the sufferer to presume that she will never walk again. She may so completely believe this that she refuses to use walking aids, to get a job or to resume any of the activities that may still be well within her grasp.

On the other hand, the ostensible absence of the disease during remission often induces the false idea of a permanent cure. Thus, remission can be dangerously threatened by the refusal to abandon obsolete world models, which then continue to determine behavior as though the disease had never occurred, or has disappeared completely — a gilt-edged invitation to relapse.

Another way of adapting to the loss of yesterday's world is to modify it, or retain at least parts of it. Even when the multiple sclerotic makes a determined effort to turn her back on the past, old forms continue to be used, expectations arise and habits of thought and action reassert themselves. Thus it seems that efforts to forget the past and dismiss the old world from one's mind are apt to fail and, indeed, there are many aspects of one world which can and, perhaps, should carry over into the next. Memories do add to our stock of solutions, but there is also the danger that blind adherence to outdated inner forms may restrict freedom of action and limit autonomous development. This is the main problem when old models are incorporated into new; we tend to build in parts that are obsolete alongside those that still have positive value.

A third way is to encapsulate some aspects of the old world. This is likely to happen if the transition has been preceded by a long period of uncertainty, as so often occurs in multiple sclerosis where diagnosis is a lengthy business leaving the individual apprehensive, distressed and, generally, fearing the worst. Then a provisional model of the world *as it may be* begins to coexist with the model of the world *as it is,* acting as an escape route if the anxiety generated by attempts to live with the reality of multiple sclerosis becomes intolerable.

Multiple sclerotics tend to hold on to the *status quo* at all costs and to avoid mastering the new tasks appropriate to a different, unwanted world. Even a global rejection of the past is somehow easier than the slow and distressing process of finding out, little by little, which elements of our old world can be retained and which must be given up. Meanwhile, our competence is greatly reduced and those around us must make allowances for our shortcomings. We need protection, reassurance, time to recoup and assistance in recreating a blueprint for the future.

In these circumstances, a fellow sufferer often constitutes some kind of system or formula through which the complexity of the private experience of being multiple sclerotic can be filtered. As a rule, the person who has recently become multiple sclerotic is preoccupied with the problem of her own future adaptation. Lacking any sound basis for prediction, her thoughts range over a variety of possibilities where she often sees herself as perpetually crippled and helpless. It is only when she meets someone in a more serious condition than herself, who appears to be coping well and cheerfully with her disability, that she is able to look at the future optimistically.

As in so many other areas, multiple sclerosis only highlights the essential elements of the human condition. Today, multiple sclerotics and nonmultiple sclerotics alike face the absolute necessity for radical change at the level of self-awareness in order to survive. Failure to achieve a realistic transition from the old to the new, whether multiple sclerotic or not, is usually due to psychic numbing.[47] This is the incapacity to feel or deal with certain kinds of experience due to the blocking or absence of inner forms of imagery that can connect with actual or potential experience. The symbolic process, involving the continual death and rebirth of inner form, the recreation of images that are more malleable, is inert. Psychic numbing is the core of being multiple sclerotic, but it also occurs whenever there is interference in the process of creating relevant inner forms.

At birth or shortly afterwards we seek a physiologic connection with this world. In maturity our quest becomes highly symbolised. It evolves from a nurturant relationship between mother and infant toward liason with other people, groups, ideas, historical forces: one or more of the many ways wherein life finds expression. Where this striving for attachment falters and fails, as it increasingly does for multiple sclerotics, we experience a sense of separation, of being cut off.

I am not a passive recipient of sensations from my life space. I create my world by reaching out to my environment. I react to my life space by moving within it, to keep it the same or to modify it. And because it is necessary to act in order to remain within this world, multiple sclerosis transforms it. There is the loss of real spaciousness and freedom and ease; the loss of poise, of infinite readiness; these are displaced by the contractions, contortions, postures of illness. Our first meanings of movement are literal; we find them in moving our bodies or some part of them through space and through time. Later movement, like our self-regulatory physiologic processes under the control of the autonomic nervous system, acquires symbolic attributes as well; these attributes have to do with development, progress and change. Now the empirical self begins to coexist with the *social* self. There is a contraction of time too, as though the consecutive frames of a film are frozen. It is inevitable, then, that with multiple sclerosis comes some measure of spatial and temporal stasis.

My immediate reaction to the diagnosis of multiple sclerosis was a sense of numbness in which physical and mental feeling was blunted. This was soon followed by distress with episodes of severe anxiety and mourning for those functions I thought were lost with the onset of the disease. The appalling magnitude of the fissures in my world which I recognised, and the voids I anticipated, made me withdraw to look back in anger at the implacable process of change that threatened to overwhelm and destroy me.

Thus multiple sclerosis is accompanied by the ultimate experience of psychic numbing. Grief is consequent upon the significant losses, a process of realisation, of making real the fact of loss. But if the concomitant psychic numbing can be overcome by mobilising appropriate forms of imagery, it may take a healthy course towards building a new, more complete and wholly satisfactory world; conversely, it is blocked or distorted by the inability to create viable imagery.

Within our internal worlds people are likely to be more important than things. Because man is a social animal who is often strongly attached to others in his life space, it is the loss of these that is the most frequent cause of major disruptions in the world of the multiple sclerotic. After changes in personal relationships, changes in loved possessions are the most obvious source of grief. These are the tools whereby we exercise our function in the world, extensions of the self which, next to our loved ones, we cherish most dearly. These linking objects can focus our attention on the world we have lost, thereby evoking appropriate grief. Similarly, imagery is an abundant source of pictures of the lost world that facilitates discussion and the necessary grief work.

Understanding multiple sclerosis means understanding a person and her rapidly changing relationship to the world. Our private experiences are the representations of an internal source of perpetual stimulation which normally evades our probings. Imaging can help the multiple sclerotic make a very direct connection with her internal state — a movement into the body. Connecting experiences in the past and in the present gives a sense of joyful recognition; this encourages the pursuit of the symbolic journey and the struggle to find meanings and patterns during phases of sometimes almost random imagery.

Really getting to grips with the base world of disease can come about by imaging situations that are disturbing and even life threatening. The power of imagery is that it brings us psychologically closer to events we are avoiding and feel the need to mask. Besides mirroring the lost world, linking objects and imagery reflect the whole set of assumptions now invalidated by being multiple sclerotic and which, as part of the internal world inaccessible to direct scrutiny, cannot readily be relinquished. By looking boldly at what we have lost, the demarcation between the world that is and the world that was becomes clearer. We can clarify our model of the world before becoming multiple sclerotic, as well as the situation that now obtains, to uncover those aspects of it that must change and those that can be retained. Ultimately we grow less afraid of the disease and are able to move more freely and creatively within the limitations it imposes.

Being multiple sclerotic reminds me of my own mortality. I may choose to deal with my fear by turning away from its source. But each time I do this I only add to my fear and miss an opportunity to adapt to the changes that are integral to this world where change is the single constant.

Self-Healing: III

The role of mind in disease is either neglected or thoroughly misunderstood by allopathic doctors. Recently, however, there are a handful who, in tune with the consciousness explosion, are beginning to accord to the human mind its central status in healing. To this minority, mind is the sole creator, there is no exception and nothing incurable. When mind and emotions are out of balance, the cells of natural immunity lose their efficiency. But just as mind out of balance destroys our natural state of general adaptation, so the mind may recreate balance and by restoring bodily homeostasis, recapture health.

We have all personally experienced the close-knit relationship between mind and body in our daily lives. When we are frightened, our body responds with an increased rate of heartbeat, more rapid breathing; we feel butterflies in our stomach and sweat excessively. This response to emergency alerts the body for action by stimulating the autonomic nervous system. There are, we know, nerve pathways between this and the pituitary and adrenal glands. The former secretes the hormones which regulate the rate of secretion to the other glands; the latter secretes steroids, which control metabolic processes, and the epinephrine, which readies us for fight or flight. Our bodies react regardless of whether the alarm is part of the world outside us or simply an image we hold in our mind.

A feeling of discomfort is a condensation of many events taking place in the body. Muscular tension clamps down blood vessels, slowing the flow of blood and keeping from the cells their essential supplies of nutrients, antibodies, hormones; also waste products accumulate around them because normal blood flow, necessary for bathing and cleansing each cell, is slowed. This produces changes in body temperature, in acid-base balance, and in the electrical fields around cells, contributing to the creation of fertile ground in which bacteria and virus can multiply. Discomfort is a state in which the empirical self (a kind of personification of the body's inborn healing abilities and self-regulatory principles) is unable to function at its best. This disharmonious state, maintained over a long period of time, is the one most conducive to illness.

Just as we have all undergone feelings of fear and other forms of excitation, so have we experienced those associated with relaxation. These more subtle feelings express many events taking place in the body. It is ease. It is harmony. It is the muscles relaxing, allowing blood to flow freely to all areas, encouraging nutrients, antibodies, hormones and white blood cells to travel to every part that needs them. The optimum temperature, acid-base balance and electrical fields can all become manifest in this state. When you create the sense of feeling good, you abandon your body to the self-regulatory processes, the empirical self, so inducing harmony. This is the state of true being wherein your inborn healing abilities can be most effective.

Thus the force in nature that tends to heal from within, the *vis medicatrix naturae,* known even in the days of Hippocrates, is present in each human body as a particular heartbeat, respiration rate, acid-base balance, the electromagnetic field of every cell. This part of you, regulating your physiology, is the empirical self. In contrast to the real self, change is integral to its existence. The natural cycling of body rhythms and functions begins sometime after conception and ends with death. Because this change is triggered by an optimal level of stress, its rate shifts from moment to moment, day to day, season to season. Personifying these self-regulatory principles is a way of showing that they are very much a part of you and that you *can* achieve control over them.

Just as there is a part of you reflecting the changes in a universal life force, there is another part that creates its own individual rates of change. This social self is a personification of that part that designs and constructs houses, invents calendars and clocks and yardsticks, and does the myriad things important to vocation, family and community life. But in its building up and tearing down the social self must always bargain with the empirical self and its principles of self-regulation — the changes, or rhythms, which throughout the course of evolution have somehow maintained the general adaptation of the human body to its biophysical environment.

The creations of the social self may be compatible with the homeostatic efforts of the empirical self. But it can also make the body, whose regulatory mechanisms are genetically linked to an era quite unlike that existing today, do things it would eschew if it were really taking the empirical self into account. Man-induced alterations and disturbances in his environment result in insults, excitants and stressors that evoke reactions unequal to the threat, or reactions so inappropriate as to be disruptive in their own right. As the years pass, the body's natural limits are strained unbearably and with increasingly devastating effect as the social self loses contact with its empirical counterpart.

Feelings of ease and dis-ease can tell you when your empirical self is being allowed sufficient freedom to maintain your body in a state of well-being. As adapted responses are transformed into maladapted ones, and you gradually become aware that your true being has been disallowed, the best way to reopen the lines of communication between social and empirical selves is through relaxation.

Since the late 1960s Dr. Herbert Benson of Harvard Medical School has studied the body's physiologic response to relaxation. He found that after twelve minutes of relaxation his subjects' oxygen consumption decreased by an average of 13 percent, their carbon dioxide production by 12 percent and their respirations from sixteen to eleven breaths per minute. These physiologic changes are called the *relaxation response*.[5]

Dr. Benson has also found that the relaxation response is

accompanied by decreased blood lactate, relatively low blood pressure, slightly increased forearm blood flow, decreased heart rates and intensification of alpha brain waves. Some fifty years ago it was discovered that the brain produces very small amounts of electricity and that these minute frequencies can be measured by electrodes placed on the outside of the head. The machine used is called an electroencephalograph and in normal people gives specific readings. These frequencies have now been subdivided and given different names.

Beta waves are produced when the person is active — looking, speaking, listening, moving about. Alpha waves depend on the individual quieting, relaxing, with eyes shut. However, it is not just a matter of stilling the body but also of emptying the mind. As so many investigators have demonstrated since then, and people from every walk of life have confirmed, this induces a conscious sense of well-being that increases self-confidence and one's powers of concentration.

The brain waves change again in sleep, when they are identified as delta waves. These vary according to the depth of unconsciousness, but change if the sleep is drug-induced. They change once more when the person is in a state of coma, deep hypnosis or trance; these are called theta waves. But these brain waves are not only evident under specific conditions. Some adults produce alpha waves even when they are active and their eyes are open. Some can produce theta waves without going into a trance, and all these frequencies vary enormously from one individual to another.

Perhaps the most important finding is that you can be trained, or *train yourself,* to get rid of your beta, or tension waves, and increase your alpha, or peace, waves. These can be vividly increased by relaxing; in true relaxation the alpha waves are a guide to how well or otherwise one is achieving this response. Dr. Benson suggests that it is the opposite of Dr. Cannon's fight or flight response. He calls it a hypometabolic state — that is, one of lowered metabolic processes — resulting from decreased autonomic system activity.

This means that you are able, in a general way, to control your own body physiology. You can do things that lower the output of the autonomic or so-called "involuntary" nervous system. This is an integrated response in that a group of general changes in the body takes place each time you relax. For hundreds of years holy men and women, Zen masters and yogis, have known that this can be done and have demonstrated the remarkable effect of mental and physical relaxation on health. The techniques they use to raise their heart rate from 80 to 300 beats per minute, or their body temperature sufficiently to melt snow, are made up of detailed images of visualisations. In short, through visualisation anyone can learn to control and use the body's own regulatory mechanisms for self-healing.

The idea that our own thoughts, our imaginations, play a decisive role in health and illness confers on us an enormous responsibility, one which we previously delegated entirely to our doctors. But the human imagination has its own properties and ongoing nature that present us with a reality even more fundamental than the sense impressions we receive from our environment. Imagery is an essential part of that reality, and the continual unfolding of imagery and the transformations of symbolism are intrinsically curative, although this function so often aborts.

Visualisations have been used for healing, both by affecting body physiology in a general way — namely, via the relaxation response — and in a specific way — that is, by increasing blood flow to one area of the body. Relaxation is the first step in gaining control over self-healing physiologic changes.

In order to relax you need to be able to distinguish tension from relaxation. Most people know when their muscles really are tense, but they usually cannot detect low levels of tension; they do not feel able to relax their muscles at will. You can become aware of the difference between tension and relaxation by tensing a muscle and then letting it go.

With your arm resting on a flat surface, raise your hand by bending it up at the wrist. With your hand raised, the muscles on top of your forearm, below the elbow, will be contracted, tense. Let your hand go limp, those muscles relax and your hand drops. The feeling of tension, of contraction, when you raise your hand is subtle. If your hand goes back too far you may be confused by a feeling of strain in the opposing muscles of your lower forearm. If at first you do not feel the upper forearm tension, alternately raise your hand in a slow, even motion and then let it go limp. Exercises like this help you become aware of tension-relaxation in any muscle of your body.

Another technique for achieving body relaxation involves autosuggestion, comprising basically a set of verbal instructions. Mentally repeat these and allow the suggestions to work by themselves. *Allowing* relaxation to take place is important. "To make good suggestions it is absolutely necessary to do it without effort . . . the use of the will . . . must be entirely put aside. One must have recourse exclusively to the imagination."[24] This is similar to the effect that Zen philosophers have referred to as "letting go."

Giving yourself a set of instructions through inner speech is fundamental to bringing your inner processes under control. The instructions need not be memorised, but you must have a sense of the meaning of words that are best suited to yourself. What you are doing is programming your own biocomputer by giving yourself a set of instructions to accomplish a particular goal.

Find a tranquil place where you will not be disturbed. Lie down with your legs uncrossed and your arms at your sides. Close your eyes, inhale slowly and deeply. Pause a moment; exhale slowly and completely. Allow your abdomen to rise and fall as you breathe. Do this several times. As you relax, your breathing becomes slow and even. Mentally say to yourself, "My feet are relaxing. They are becoming more and more relaxed. My feet feel heavy." Rest for a moment. Repeat the same suggestions for your ankles. Rest again. In the same way, relax your lower legs, then your thighs, pausing to feel the sensations of relaxation in your muscles. Relax your pelvis. Rest. Relax abdomen. Rest. Relax the muscles of your back. Rest. Relax your chest. Rest. Relax your fingers; hands; forearms; upper arms; shoulders. Rest. Relax your neck. Rest. Relax your jaw, allowing it to drop. Relax your tongue; cheeks, eyes. Rest.

Relax your forehead and the top of your head. Now just rest. Allow your whole body to relax.

You are now in a calm relaxed state which you can deepen by counting backwards. Breath in; as you exhale slowly, say to yourself, "Ten. I am feeling very relaxed." Inhale again, and as you exhale, repeat mentally, "Nine. I am feeling more relaxed." Breathe. "Eight. I am feeling even more relaxed." "Seven. Deeper and more relaxed." "Six. Even more . . ." Five (pause). Four (pause). Three (pause). Two (pause). One (pause). Zero (pause).

You are now at a deeper and more relaxed level of awareness where your body feels healthy, your mind peaceful and open. It is a level at which you can experience images in your mind more clearly and vividly than ever before. You can stay in this relaxed state as long as you like. To return to ordinary consciousness, mentally say, "I am now going to move. When I count to three, I will raise my left hand and stretch my fingers. I will then feel relaxed, happy and strong, ready to continue my everyday activities."

Develop your own technique of relaxing because, as with everything else, the same methods do not suit everyone equally well. The basic principles are simple: make yourself as comfortable as possible; use a suitable chair with a headrest if lying down is inclined to make you fall asleep. Practice your relaxation at least twice a day. The habit of always using the same room is helpful. Silence is vitally important, so exclude all sound. Take off your shoes and loosen any tight band or restriction round your neck and waistline. Be sure to be warm enough for the whole period of quietness. Dogs and cats, however still, are much more often a distraction than a help, though many people have a relationship with their pets such that they can enhance the atmosphere rather than spoil it. Just be sure, though, that you are not allergic to animal dander!

Each time you relax, by whichever method, you will find it easier and relax more deeply. People experience the sensation of relaxation as tingling, radiating or pulsing. They feel warmth or coolness, heaviness or a floating sensation. When they have followed a method of relaxation several times, they may be able to relax deeply just by breathing in and out and allowing themselves to go.

Deep relaxation clears your mind and removes muscular tension which can be distracting. To visualise effectively, you must also be able to concentrate, to fix your mind on one thought or image and to hold it there. People seldom realise how little control they have over their own thoughts. You can test this by trying to concentrate only on counting your breaths for a few minutes; you will probably immediately find other thoughts going through your mind which make you lose track of counting. To use the breath-counting exercise to build concentration, just return to the count each time an intrusive thought enters your mind. Cut off the thought in mid-air, as it were. This prevents you from becoming enmeshed in a train of thoughts that does not pertain to the count.

All our self-regulatory processes, our heartbeat and respiration, everything that makes up our empirical self, functions by the grace of our immune system, for this is committed to the defence of life itself. Operating entirely at the level of physics and chemistry the wildest flight of fancy could not have foreseen that we and our auto-selves — a personification of our antibodies, T and B lymphocytes, complement, granulocytes and macrophages — would someday meet.

But in this last quarter of the twentieth century the conscious control of our auto-self does not seem far-fetched. We know that how we feel affects the functioning of our empirical self, once considered way beyond our thoughts and emotions. And now we find that the hormones circulating in our blood, increasing or decreasing in amount in harmony with how we feel, individually and specifically affect the three different cell types of our auto-self regulating the movements and functioning of our macrophages and our killer T-cells, as well as the antibody producing abilities of our B lymphocytes.

Stress influences the auto-self in various ways, activating the pituitary and adrenal glands, causing involution of the thymus and bringing about anamnestic reactions (reaction of recalling, defined as the enhancement of antibody titre) which, in turn, reactivate pre-existent immune responses. There is a volume of evidence on the effect of stress on different immune processes in animals. Some are inhibited, but generally, susceptibility to infection is increased. Nothing comparable on immune reactions in humans exists, and very few observations; although we are told that in military personnel, malaria often "appeared after the added stress of surgery and anesthesia, including minor procedures";[85] in man, "surgical trauma is associated with a number of temporary deficits in the immune system that might conceivably lead to increased susceptibility to infection or tumour spread";[95] and in miners, prolonged exposure to work stress caused "a significant decrease of all three classes of Ig. In the group exposed for a shorter time only the IgG decreased significantly."[85] These reports come largely from Russian investigators, but in the West W. J. Fessel demonstrated that mental stress alone produces a rise in a person's circulating IgM.[85] McClary, an Australian researcher, found that the onset of systemic lupus eyrthematosus (SLE) often followed a major life stress situation. SLE is a bizarre autoimmune disease caused, apparently, by DNA escaping from a few cells into the bloodsteam. Once there it is read by the immune system as foreign, and antibodies are made against it. The DNA, coupled to the body's anti-DNA antibodies, is usually deposited in the kidneys.

But at a medical centre in the Southwest of the United States, a small step for man and a genuinely giant step for mankind is underway, quietly, without undue fuss or publicity. There a specialist in the treatment of cancer and himself a victim of ulcer disease, sensed that the fault might be *his*, not his stomach's, that his suffering was something he might be responsible for, something he was doing, or not doing, to his Self. He wondered too, about other diseases, and about the responsibility of others for their own illnesses. In the early seventies, he decided that the time was ripe to try to make contact with his auto-self.

Dr. Carl Simonton is a rare breed of doctor, one who truly understands the real nature of the physician's task: to help the body do what it has learned so well to do on its own during its eternal struggle for survival — to heal itself. In addition to the conventional medical treatments for cancer sufferers, he also instructs his patients about their bodies. He explains what their antibodies are, what molecules look like, where they are made. He tells patients about their immune systems, and how the immune system originally tried to combat the first tumour cells, attempting to destroy them before they could get a foothold. He tells them about their white cells, their T and B lymphocytes, about the messenger lymphocytes in their circulation, and about the transformation to killer cells. He makes sure patients know how the immune system works and how, in their own particular cases, the immune system, despite its heroic efforts, has been beaten back and finally overwhelmed by the cancer cells.

He explains about radiation therapy, the cobalt machine and anti-cancer drugs; how some tumour cells will be killed, others weakened; how the massacre will release cancer antigens into their bloodstream, stimulating the production of more anti-cancer antibodies and more killer lymphocytes so that the immune system can take up its defences once more.

He describes how the white cells and macrophages will pour over the radiated tumour, penetrate the irradiated, drug-filled malignant mass and begin to devour the cancer cells. He shows the cancer sufferers their X-rays with the masses in their stomachs or chests so they know exactly what they are up against. He makes absolutely certain each person understands his own anatomy and physiology, and his disease. When they do, when they are quite clear about the path over which their cure could come, when they know how healing can be effected, Dr. Simonton begins to teach them to meditate.

He encourages them to visualise their tumours and then to concentrate on the battle between themselves and their disease. He tells them to turn in upon themselves, to think of their antibodies, to will them to make their way toward their tumours, to force their killer lymphocytes to take up a more lethal attack on their cancer cells. In short, he encourages them to actively participate in the defence of their own bodies, to bend their minds unremittingly to the task of person survival. Finally, just before they cease meditating, he asks them to visualise themselves well and healthy.

Bob Gilley, a forty-year-old executive with cancer worked with Dr. Simonton using visualisation. Before seeing him, Gilley's survival was estimated at 30 percent. Of his work with visualisation Gilley says, "I'd begin to visualise my cancer as I saw it my mind's eye. I'd make a game of it. The cancer would be a snake, a wolverine or some vicious animal. The cure, white husky dogs by the millions. It would be a confrontation of good and evil. I'd envision the dogs grabbing the cancer and shaking it, ripping it to shreds. The forces of good would win. The cancer would shrink from a big snake to a little snake and then disappear. Then the white army of dogs would lick up the residue and clean my abdominal cavity until it was spotless."[8] Gilley did this three times a day for ten to fifteen minute intervals. After six weeks of meditation, an examination revealed his tumour had shrunk by 75 percent. After two months Gilley had a cancer scan. There was no trace of the disease in his body. Simonton has since achieved similar success in other cases with far worse prognoses. In one instance the sufferer who had only between 5 to 10 percent chance to live could be released after a few weeks, cured, and with no side-effects.

Simonton is also trying to educate people, including the sufferer's whole family, to look to cancer without dread and to know that help can be found in their own attitude of mind and that they are *not* helpless. He is accumulating evidence on why and how the mind can affect cancer cells. He feels that the effects of mental tension in the body is underrated and that people go for years unaware that they are damaging the normal cells of their body in this way. He believes they learn to accept stress as normal, to live with it, not recognising it as connected with their health problems. The body will always heal itself, given a chance, and the deep relaxation of meditation provides this chance. Visualisation might be only a mystical concept were it not visible on recorded alpha waves, so that full relaxation and concentration of mind prepares the body for return to its natural state of general adaptation.

Simonton's technique deals with a process: visualising cancer cells being carried off by white blood cells. However, with multiple sclerosis where the sites of the lesions in the central nervous system are uncertain, we have to deal with a final state: visualising oneself recovered and healthy.

To succeed with your own healing, you must believe, above all, that you are *not* helpless. Then, *relax*. Next imagine actual healing processes occurring in your body. There are various sources upon which you can draw to create clear images of healing. If you invent your own, choose ones which describe, *by your own interpretation,* the basic healing processes: erasing bacteria or viruses; building new cells to replace damaged myelin (refer to Figs. 1 and 2, page 8); making sore areas comfortable; draining edemous tissue; releasing pressure from tight areas; bringing blood to areas that need nutriment, as Professor Russell suggests; making areas that are wet drier; bringing energy to areas that are fatigued; bringing the capacity for movement to areas that have lost it, perhaps by attaching imaginary strings that you can manipulate in order to move and control recalcitrant fingers and feet.

After imagining the healing processes taking place, and as you feel these processes beginning, imagine the way the central

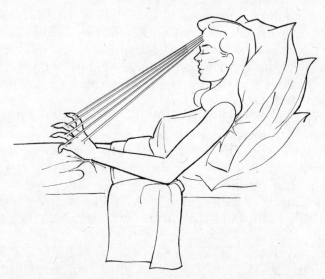

Figure 3. Imaging cords to manipulate paralysed fingers.

nervous system looks and feels in its completely healed state. Use visualisation with the same regularity demanded by any other healing method, such as drugs or physical therapy. You are freeing inborn healing abilities to do their work. No healing can occur without them, but you can do many things to strengthen them, encourage them and release them.

In some circumstances the general nature of final-state visualisations allows the healing process to take place more naturally than the more directed, process visualisations. Visualising a healed state can involve simply seeing yourself as radiantly healthy. Close your eyes. Relax your whole body by whatever method works best for you. Then let your ideas of disease symptoms become bubbles in your consciousness. Now imagine that these bubbles are being flown out of your mind, out of your body, out of your consciousness by a breeze which draws them away from you, far into the distance, until you no longer see them or feel them. Watch them disappear over the horizon.

Now imagine that you are in a place you love: beach, mountain, desert, wherever you feel alive, comfortable, healthy. Imagine that the area around you is filled with bright, clear light. Allow it to flow into your body, making you brighter and filling you with all the vital energy of true being.

Every method devised for the acquisition of self-awareness gives a great deal of consideration to establishing control over the body, which is the first step in gaining control over the conscious self.

Self-awareness is closely allied to our ability to direct our attention. At any time, we may find ourselves occupying any one of our selves. The main criterion for identifying these different selves is the quality of our attention. Most of the time it is captured by outside forces — sounds, colours, etc. — or else by forces inside of us — fears, worries, etc. Without attention, or with attention wandering in this way, we are in the mechanical self.

However, there is always the possibility of freely and deliberately directing our attention to something entirely of our own choosing. With our attention attracted by the subject of reflection (for example our visualisations) and kept there, we are in the empirical self. With the attention attracted by the subject of observation and held there by thought we are in the conscious self; whereas when it is directed to the subject by will, we are in the pure or existential self. It is the shiftless moving of our attention that renders us incompetent and less than fully human.

Our circumstances are not merely the facts of life as we meet them but also, and even more, the ideas in our minds. Thus it is impossible to gain any control over circumstances without first controlling our ideas, and the breath counting exercise quickly shows how difficult that is. The most important and universal teaching of all the religions is that *vipassana*, the clarity of vision, can be attained only if you are able to put the conscious self in its place; it must remain silent when so ordered and act only when given a definite and specific task.

The Christian method of shifting the conscious self to where it belongs and keeping it there is an inner prayer, the "prayer of the heart." Brought to perfection in the Greek and Russian Orthodox Churches, its essence is "standing before God with the mind in the heart." The prayer of the heart, normally the Jesus Prayer (consisting in English of these words: "Lord Jesus Christ, Son of God, have mercy upon me, a sinner"), is endlessly repeated by the mind *in the heart,* and this vitalises, moulds and reforms the whole person. Its effect has been explained by Theophan the Recluse: "In order to keep the mind on one thing by the use of a short prayer, it is necessary to preserve attention and so lead it into the heart: for so long as the mind remains in the head, where thoughts jostle one another, it has no time to concentrate on one thing. But when attention descends into the heart, it attracts all the powers of the soul and body into one point there. This concentration of all human life in one place is immediately reflected in the heart by a special sensation that is the beginning of future warmth. This sensation, faint at the beginning, becomes gradually stronger, firmer, deeper. At first only tepid, it grows into warm feeling and concentrates the attention upon itself. And so it comes about that, whereas in the initial stages the attention is

kept in the heart by an effort of will, in due course this attention, by its own vigour, gives birth to warmth in the heart.
This warmth then holds the attention without special effort.
From this, the two go on supporting one another, and must
remain inseparable; because dispersion of attention cools the
warmth, and diminishing warmth weakens attention."[15]

The assertion that the endless repetition, silently, of a short
sequence of words leads to a spiritual result, represented by
physical sensations of spiritual warmth is likely to be regarded
by many as the surest sign of psychosis. This is because
Western civilisation, clad tight in the garb of technology,
cannot grasp that at the human level of being the invisible is of
infinitely greater power than all the visible manifestations of
the physical world. Our technologic competence is breathtaking and our bemusement, ignorance and downright incompetence in respect of essentially human concerns even more so.*

In his book *Mysticism and Philosophy*, W. T. Stace, a professor of philosophy at Princeton University asks, "What
bearing, if any, does what is called "mystical experience" have
upon the more important problems of philosophy?"[93] He
points out that there is no doubt that the basic psychologic
facts about the "introvertive type of mystical experience" are, in
essence, "the same all over the world in all cultures, religions,
places and ages." They are, he says, "so extraordinary and
paradoxical that they are bound to strain belief when suddenly
sprung upon anyone who is not prepared for them. Suppose,"
he continues, "that one should stop up the inlets of the physical senses so that no sensations could reach consciousness . . . There seems to be no *a priori* reason why a man bent
on the goal . . . should not, by acquiring sufficient concentration and mental control, exclude all physical sensations from

---

*Iatrogenesis is preeminently a failure of the human imagination: a radical failure to
conceive in human terms the meaning of contemporary medical technology leading to
the embrace, as a means of salvation, of that which most seriously threatens our health.

Iatrogenesis is a peculiar twentieth century disease of power. Man has always
attached deep emotion to his tools, but never more so than now. Tragically, the
precarious sense of his own mortality bred by the proliferation of technology, as well as
his denial of death, makes him peculiarly vulnerable to aberrations of the scientific-
rational image.

his consciousness.

"Suppose that, after having got rid of all sensations, one should go on to exclude from consciousness all sensuous images and then all abstract thoughts, reasoning processes, volitions, and other particular contents; what would then be left of consciousness? There would be no mental content whatever but rather a complete emptiness, vacuum, void."[93]

This is, of course, the aim of those who wish to study their inner life: the exclusion of all disturbing influences emanating from the senses or from the conscious self. Professor Stace, however, becomes deeply puzzled. "One would suppose *a priori* that consciousness would then entirely lapse and one would fall asleep or become unconscious. But the introvertive mystics, thousands of them all over the world, unanimously assert that they have attained to this complete vacuum of particular mental contents, but what then happens is quite different from a lapse into unconsciousness. On the contrary, what emerges is a state of *pure* consciousness, 'pure' in the sense that it is not the consciousness *of* any empirical content. It has no content except itself."

"Our normal everyday consciousness always has objects, or images, or even our own feelings or thoughts perceived introspectively. Suppose then that we obliterate all objects physical or mental. *When the self is not engaged in apprehending objects it becomes aware of itself.* The self itself emerges . . ."[93]

Professor Stace's view corroborates the central teaching of the great religions which urge man to open himself to the Self or Divine Power that dwells within him; to transcend consciousness by self-awareness. Only by liberating ourselves from the tyranny of the senses and of thought by withdrawing attention from the things seen to give it to the things unseen, can we accomplish this awakening.

Self-Healing: IV

Homo non proprie humanus sed superhumanus est.
To be properly human, you must go beyond the merely human.

No matter how much the subject that says "I," the Self, is weighed down by being multiple sclerotic, there is always the possibility of self-assertion and a rising above circumstances. We can all achieve a measure of control over our environment and thereby our lives. There are no definable limits to our possibilities, even though in the state of being multiple sclerotic, as in anything else, there are practical limitations that restrain us.

In many ways the multiple sclerotic is an object, dependent, slave to the caprice of the disease. Aware of this we must again use our imagination, as sick and healthy peoples everywhere have always done, to complete our development as human beings. Having assumed control over all our other me's to enhance inner coherence and strength, and having begun our exploration of the self, we conceive a Being, wholly active, sovereign, autonomous: a person above all merely human persons; in no way an object; above all circumstances and contingencies, entirely in control of everything — a personal God, the Unmoved Mover.

Somewhere along the evolutionary path we had, of necessity, to become less acutely aware of our spiritual roots so that we could find our feet. We lost our souls in order to gain our minds, so to speak. However, absolute independence — even if it were possible — would deprive us of direction or purpose, and of stability. Some contact with whatever forces guide our evolution must be maintained. In ancient civilisations myths and mythologies and religious teachings were the symbolic means whereby such links were forged. Through these man experienced himself as existing on earth, brought there by forces and powers he variously called gods, God or nature. As the centuries went by, his connections with them weakened, as slowly, very slowly, he learned to make his own way.

Evolution occurs in epochs, and the past three hundred years or so has seen the flowering of man's ability to think, particularly about his physical world. The result is modern science and a technologic euphoria. The main theme of the sci-tech myth that permeates our thinking about nature is one of conquest. We are fair set to vanquish nature, disease, pain and even death. Willy-nilly, fate will be outwitted. So we transmute one human experience after another into a technical problem in order to bring it under our firm control; any that resist are ignored or denied. In this imperceptible manner do we robber barons divest all our experience of personal or intrinsic meaning.

The sci-tech myth tells us that the universe began as a vast array of hot hydrogen atoms, a sort of primeval sun. Then by a series of complex cosmologic processes there evolved more complex atoms and the physical universe of galaxies and, at a comparatively late stage within this, there came into being our solar system.

This, it is said, started as a hot mass of gaseous atoms from which the sun, the planets, our earth and moon subsequently separated out. Then by more complex processes, there came about on earth organic molecules which somehow gave rise to life, at first as elementary cells. By further unknown processes these gave rise to form and function in plants and animals and, finally, man. And then within man himself consciousness (the ability to understand what is taking place in and around us) came into being.

Hydrogen atoms cannot themselves decide to embark on an evolutionary path whereby they develop into a universe, and a star system, and into conscious human beings; some force or forces must operate to bring these developments about — indeed forces are necessary to bring the material world of hydrogen atoms into existence in the first place.

But even if we knew what the nature of these forces was, we still do not know how and why *they* came into being. Why are we in an evolving universe? We could equally well have found ourselves in one that was not evolving, or in one that was doing so according to some other pattern.

Nowadays most of us assume that questions like these cannot be given an objective answer: even if there is a pattern we could not find it, so that it is all a matter of "belief" or "faith." Thus the sci-tech myth evaporates into thin air just at the point where the fundamental issues of human life begin. More important, however, as descriptive science, it becomes unscientific and illegitimate precisely when it begins to indulge in comprehensive explanatory theories, like evolutionism, which can be neither verified nor falsified by experiment. Such a theory itself requires an act of faith that many biologists and other scientists with impeccable credentials have refused to make, simply because, as psychiatrist Karl Stern observes, ". . . such a view of cosmogenesis is crazy. And I do not mean crazy in the sense of slangy invective, but rather in the technical meaning of psychotic. Indeed such a view has much in common with certain aspects of schizophrenic thinking."[94]

E. F. Schumacher comments on the matter with his accustomed discernment: "Evolutionism as currently presented has no basis in science. It is not science; it is science fiction, even a kind of hoax. It is a hoax that has succeeded too well and has imprisoned modern man in what looks like an irreconcilable conflict between 'science' and 'religion' . . . Evolutionism, purporting to explain all and everything solely and exclusively by natural selection for adaptation and survival, is the most extreme product of the materialistic utilitarianism of the nineteenth century. The inability of twentieth century thought to rid itself of this imposture is a failure that may well cause the collapse of Western civilisation."[80]

Yet the era that started about 1600 with Francis Bacon has nurtured many myths besides, the majority of which leave us with a vague sense that the material affluence on which sci-tech's prestige rests is not worthy as an end in itself. Have we forgotten altogether about the quality of life? Material and economic problems are no longer basic. We have the knowledge and expertise to lavish on ourselves an unprecedented standard of material well-being. But we know nothing about how to use this knowledge to promote human happiness. We do not know how to enable people to live and work together in harmony, so that our technologic skills are used effectively and efficiently. Nor do we know how the wealth spawned by industrialism can be equitably distributed. Least of all do we see that these are ethical and spiritual problems that no amount of manipulation of world economies will ever solve.

The crushing emphasis on material existence has led to the

neglect of our spiritual well-being. The decade of the sixties overflowed with bizarre efforts to find something — anything — that would bridge the gap between these disparate aspects. With the Aquarian Age dawned a bright new image of man and society. Soon youth from all social strata began to drop out. They sought their own authenticity, revolted by our hypocrisies. They saw too that alienation, the divorce of man from his ecosystem, and not cancer or multiple sclerosis or heart failure, is the real terminal disease of mankind.

They expressed their protest in their life-style, became hippies, flower children, Jesus freaks, lived in communes, smoked pot, spoke their own hip language, ate macrobiotic food, professed universal love and practiced free sex. Despite many strange manifestations, this spontaneous movement of dissent, self-indulgence and spiritual quest was the seed of the consciousness explosion: the overt expressions of an inward journey. Youth today are seeking mystically, magically, pharmacologically, to establish a personal, covert world of purpose, power and coherence to compensate for the chaos and desolation of the world we bequeathed to them.

The psychedelic drugs were attractive in that they swiftly paved the way to a richer inner experience; however, they also destroyed clarity of thought. Meditation, married to a clear evaluation of the insights it encouraged, seemed to offer a safer avenue for personal exploration. But many meditational paths, while sometimes leading to spiritual ecstasy, are really divertissements, far from the Way, the Truth and the Life. In their strangely mindless flight from heartless materialism youth forgot to monitor its spiritual adventures with the lucidity and precision of thought that is our hard-won contribution to human evolution. No one, until E. F. Schumacher, noted the crucial difference between consciousness and a consciousness aware of itself, the distinction so elaborately explored in Jean Piaget's technical works. Youth in consequence has not yet mastered the art of separating the spiritual from the occult.

So began a fresh search for a realistic metaphysics that could restore the spiritual connection between man and his gods, that could reconnect man with reality and those unknown sources of energy at higher levels of being, taking us another small step along the stony evolutionary path. Change is imperative if we are to survive the sci-tech tempest, and the requisite change is at the human level of being. We have tried institutional changes and ideological changes and behavioral changes without noticeable effect. The problems presented by a runaway technology have not yielded one inch to any of these attacks. Our last survival strategy, our only hope is to become able to transcend the conscious self to reach the level of self-awareness, for "the conscious self is as ignorant of spiritual things as is a beast of rational things," and must always remain so.

There have been other, earlier attempts to change at the level of being in many spheres of human life and thought. Near the beginning of the sci-tech age erudite men like William Blake foresaw the pitfalls in the course being laid. G. B. Shaw was only one who did his formidable best for health by trying to counteract the public's blind faith in the efficiency as well as in the integrity of the medical profession. Did he not roundly condemn compulsory vaccination and praise the wisdom of his older contemporaries who took care to consult doctors qualified before 1860, when the germ theory of disease took root? But what impact did his plays really have? Not much, evidently. At the time Shaw wrote his amusing tirades, however, the dangers to mankind of the scientific-rational image were very far from the purview of the man in the street. They have become obvious only in the past twenty years or so. "Until now mankind has withstood the ravages of even present-day medicine, but never underestimate its power to exterminate" — a chilling remark from an unremembered source.

People today are aware, in a general sense, that the urban-industrial-scientific-technologic experiment has created more problems than it can solve. As the 1972 Club of Rome's Project Report on the predicament of mankind made us all aware, there are limits to growth, and if the world's major industrial powers continue to pursue economic growth and to foster an ethic based on ever-increasing production and consumption of goods, the planet's resources will rapidly be depleted and the environment irremediably polluted. But people are not aware, unless they read Ivan Illich, that there are also limits to medicine: the medical profession has been called the greatest hazard to health today and iatrogenic diseases the fastest spreading epidemic in the western world.

The complexity of the sick person's environment grows daily. Each year the potency and the number of drugs increases at a rate that strains the clinician's capacity to grasp their significance and modes of action. Add to this the different forms of radiant energy, catheters and instruments capable of exploring almost every vessel and body orifice, contrast media and biopsies, and the picture still is not complete. These resources differ from drugs in that by themselves they are more or less inert — a notion that clinical ecology seriously challenges — requiring activation by the doctor who may abuse them because of lack of skill and wisdom. But all are the tools and products of two decades of medical progress that is unprecedented in mankind's history. They are a powerful arsenal with much that is beneficial, but which also has considerable potential for harm. The mushrooming of this inherent character of chemotherapeutic agents and of diagnostic and therapeutic instrumentation has introduced a truly formidable dimension in the causation of human diseases. No longer need the doctor play second fiddle to the virus, the bacillus and the parasite. The drugs and investigatory procedures available to the doctor almost guarantee that our bodies will also be irremediably polluted. In fact, we are now far too clever to be able to survive without wisdom.

A shift in awareness, an image change, essential if we are to use the fruits of the sci-tech revolution wisely, quintessential if the doctor is to deploy his arsenal so that its good is maximised and its harm minimised, depends partly on our basing our lives and social practices on a deeper and broader truth than the one we are committed to now. Most of our problems arise from our values and priorities which, in turn, derive from a view of man, nature and cosmos that is partial, unidimensional, shortsighted and, in the last analysis, simply untrue. To create "a steady state of economic and ecological equilibrium" the Club of Rome's Report concluded, will require "A Copernican revolution of the mind and if the human species is to survive man must explore himself — his goals and values — as much as the world he seeks to change."[53]

But it depends also on recognising that the creation of the new world begins in man himself. It starts with the evolution of inner space, the scene of freedom now usurping outer space in importance, formed by the powers of life, consciousness and self-awareness. Dr. Maurice Nicoll sees it this way: "At first all is darkness: then light appears and is separated from the darkness. By this light we understand a form of consciousness to which our ordinary consciousness is, by comparison, darkness. This light has constantly been equated with truth and freedom. Inner perception of oneself, of one's invisibility, is the beginning of light."[64]

Scientific efforts, methodologically restricted to the material aspects of the universe, can never obtain evidence of the existence of levels of being higher than man himself. Conversely, prophets, sages and saints, in different languages but with virtually one voice, declare that there are levels of being above that of humanity, and that we can reach these higher levels, provided that we allow our reason to be guided by faith. Faith is a fundamental presupposition about our world directing our intellect to an understanding of the higher levels; it is *not* as the sci-tech myth would have it, opposed to the intellect and therefore something to be derided, scoffed at and rejected out of hand.

As far as St. Augustine is concerned, faith is the heart of the matter. "*Faith tells us what there is to understand;* it purifies the heart, and so allows reason to profit from discussion; it enables reason to arrive at an understanding of God's revelation. In short, when St. Augustine speaks of understanding, he always has in mind the product of a rational activity for which faith prepares the way."[34]

Faith opens "the eye of truth" as the Buddhists say, producing insight and comprehension, as opposed to the opinions arrived at by thinking. "Recognising the poverty of philosophical opinions" says the Buddha, "not adhering to any of them seeking the truth, *I saw.*"[97] The process of mobilising the various powers possessed by man, gradually, organically, is described in a Buddhist text: "One cannot, I say, attain supreme knowledge all at once; only by a gradual training, a gradual action, a gradual unfolding, does one attain perfect knowledge. In what manner? A man comes, moved by confidence; having come, he joins; having joined, he listens; listening, he receives the doctrine; having received the doctrine, he remembers it; he examines the sense of the things remembered; from examining the sense, the things are approved of; having approved, desire is born; he ponders; pondering, he eagerly trains himself; and eagerly training himself, he mentally realises the highest truth itself and, penetrating it by means of wisdom, *he sees.*"[52]

This is the process of developing the instrument capable of seeing and thus understanding the truth that does not merely inform the mind but liberates the self. It means systematic work to keep in contact with and develop towards higher levels than those of ordinary life or of the state of being multiple sclerotic with all its losses and pain and suffering. It means, in short, *religio*.

Biologic Dietetics

The exploration of *any* matter of medical significance is predominantly analytic. But nowhere is investigation by analysis more thorough or detailed than in the field of nutrition and that of its practical application, dietetics.

The foundations of modern analytic nutrition were laid by two chemists: Frenchman Antoine-Laurent Lavoisier and a German, J. Liebig. Lavoisier discovered that, in essence, respiration is the intake of oxygen and the output of carbon dioxide involving a kind of combustion. His work made possible a quantitative examination of the processes of metabolism together with the classification of foodstuffs in terms of their combustion value in calories. Liebig developed the modern methods of organic analysis and his most eminent pupil, Voit, the principles and techniques of calorimetry. Since then the stock-in-trade of nutritionists has been calories, protein, fat, carbohydrate and other analytic constituents of an individual's twenty-four-hour food intake. Most subsequent advances have taken the form of an ever more fractional analysis of this general intake.

The fractional approach to the daily diet, irrespective of the specific foods comprising it, has almost completely eclipsed medical interest in the overall effects of given foods. For instance, food allergy has been relegated to near oblivion. The greatest single failing of analytic diet therapy is the unfortunate conclusion that specific foods, such as wheat, corn, milk, egg, etc., are not implicated in a wide range of physical and mental symptoms. Although there is limited recognition that uncommonly eaten foods are important in isolated cases, there is complete ignorance of the fact that essentially addictive behavior actually exists to everyday foods and that these masked allergies are by far the more common and serious occurrence. Indeed, traditionally trained doctors generally ridicule the very possibility of food-related chronic illness.

The apparent reasons for this failure to diagnose allergic responses to common foodstuffs are as follows:

1. The lack of recognition of food allergy as a major cause of chronic illness.

2. The investigation of food allergy by means of skin tests with food extracts and reliance on the results of such local reactions constitute inadequate diagnostic procedures for detecting food sensitivity.

3. The preconception that the food allergy problem revolves around wheat, milk and eggs plus the routine use of basic types of elimination diets which inevitably permit the inclusion of one or more addictive foods.

4. In the case of sugars, the acceptance of allergy to corn sugar per se, but the rejection of the allergenicity of dextrose on the basis that it is a normally occurring bodily monosaccharide resulting from the metabolism of disaccharides. This view ignores the intake of exogenous dextrose derived from the hydrolysis of cornstarch as a foreign substance capable of eliciting allergic-type responses.

5. The ease with which many allergenics induce and perpet-

uate specifically adapted or addicted (masked) states allays suspicion regarding causative foods.

6. The fact that, until recently, the only diagnostic procedure able to demonstrate these cause and effect relationships was the individual food ingestion test. This test, dependent upon the complete avoidance of specific foods for a minimum of four days prior to testing, is a major obstacle because of the difficulty of being certain that abstinence has been complete.

Diet therapy in multiple sclerosis is, like all the other forms, a source of heated controversy. Studies of the geographical distribution of the disease led to theories about the role of dietetic factors. Particular attention has been paid to the relative quantities of saturated and unsaturated fatty acids in the daily diet. *Lancet* reports that the fatty tissue of the brain is greatly altered when the diet is altered. That is, a change from one kind of fat to another can have a positive effect on the health of the brain, and hence the nerves. Eating the wrong kind at some critical stage of physical development may even be linked etiologically to multiple sclerosis in later life. For instance, human breast milk contains fats, 8 percent of which are unsaturated. Cow's milk contains almost none of these. However, a baby fed on formula based on cow's milk may not be missing out on linoleic acid, but on vitamin E. It has even been suggested that vitamin E deficiency may be associated with the sudden unexpected death syndrome in infants. Because of this, in New Zealand formulas based on cow's milk, and presumably enriched with linoleic acid, are supplemented with vitamin E.

Amongst other evidence adduced in favour of the low-fat theory is the incidence of multiple sclerosis in the fishing communities of Norway, which is low compared with that in the agricultural areas; in South Africa, where it was presumed that the diet of the population as a whole is very low in saturated fatty acids, the disease is relatively rare; and the attack rate was high in persons suddenly changing from a low to a high fat diet after the migratory changes preceding, during and following World War II.

Dr. Swank,[99,100,101] in particular, has always emphasized that high-fat diets are an important etiologic factor and that a diet low in fat favourably influences the clinical course of the disease. On the other hand, critics of the low-fat theory point out that the Norwegian figures and those dealing with post-war migrants are open to doubt. Moreover, the South African figures neglect entirely the low incidence (until recently) of multiple sclerosis amongst white South Africans whose diet is certainly as rich in saturated fats as that in any other country in the world.

The fatty acid theory received a boost from biochemical studies indicating a change in the relative proportions of saturated and unsaturated fatty acids in the brain lipids of multiple sclerotics. The further discovery that sufferers had a significantly lower percentage of linoleic acid in their blood, the percentage being lowest amongst those who were experiencing acute episodes, lent further support to this theory. However, other investigators have been able to detect only minor differences in whole brain and myelin samples from multiple sclerotic and nonmultiple sclerotics. Furthermore, reference is rarely made to the fact that the decreased levels of linoleic acid in serum during acute phases is by no means specific to multiple sclerosis, but appears to be a nonspecific response to increased medical stress in general.

Subsequent clinical studies led to linoleate supplements being added to the diets of a small group of multiple sclerotics. The therapeutic regimen worked out by Dr. Millar consists of 30 ml of sunflower seed oil emulsion (containing 8.6 g of linoleic acid) given twice daily, made up to a specific formula.[56]

The sunflower seed oil diet also recommends a cut in the intake of animal (saturated) fats and an increase in the intake of vegetable (unsaturated) fats. While the two main elements of this diet, sunflower seed oil and avoidance of animal fats remain constant, the oil can be taken in different ways. The most usual is in liquid form obtainable, like any other oil, from supermarkets, chemists, grocers; the other is capsules similar in composition to the ordinary oil but more concentrated. Taking six or so of these capsules daily is often preferred to the liquid equivalent, irrespective of camouflage by orange or lemon juice. Naudicelle,® available in the United Kingdom, is also a capsule in concentrate form; it contains both the important linoleic acid plus gamma-linolenic acid, which is a stage nearer the natural conversion that takes place in our bodies before the production of structured fat. The combination of these two ingredients render Naudicelle unique, but its value is still widely debated.

Dr. Millar was understandably cautious about his conclusions regarding the linoleate supplements. He did report that the severity of relapses was less; they were of shorter duration; and their frequency was less in his treated cases. The supplementation in no way abolishes relapses, but the relapse rate per person per year in his trial was 0.54 amongst those treated as compared with 0.76 among the untreated group. Criticisms of Dr. Millar's experiment are summed up by the comment that it is "inadequate as evidence of a beneficial effect." Nevertheless, many multiple sclerotics — perhaps the majority — regularly swallow often large quantities of sunflower seed oil (active principle: linoleic acid) daily, presumably in the belief that linoleate supplementation *is* beneficial because it can rectify a low linoleic acid level. What sufferers seem not to realise is the limited success of Millar's regimen may be a reflection of something far more profound: immunosuppression.

We know from experiments with animals that their lipid status can affect an autoimmune process: that is, PUFAs (in cell membranes or in body fluids) may exercise an immunoregulatory function. Mertin argues that PUFAs act *in vivo* to inhibit the activity of cells of the immune system; when the levels of PUFAs are reduced, as in EFA-deficient animals, the activity of the immune system increases in consequence.[54] As part of the immunoregulatory system, PUFAs inhibit cellular mechanisms at high and enhance them at low concentrations. Possibly, therefore, an increase in linoleate serum level has an immunosuppressive effect, presumably damping the attack by sensitised lymphocytes upon the nervous system. Field has shown that linoleic and another EFA, arachidonic acid, do indeed significantly inhibit the antigen-induced human lymphocyte reaction to specific antigens. These positive results are interesting; more important, however, they carry far-reaching implications for therapy. For example, PUFAs in their role as immunoinhibitors have been used successfully to treat eczema.

The EFAs act as precursors of prostaglandins. These fatty acids, whose existence in the body is remarkably ephemeral, are among the most potent of all known biologic materials, producing marked effects in extremely small doses. In general, these are based on certain broad powers: regulation of the activity of smooth muscles, of secretion, including some endocrine-gland secretions, or of blood flow. Through these actions they are capable of affecting many aspects of human physiology.

Prostaglandins are synthesized in the body from certain fatty acids. One common EFA precursor is arachidonic acid. The main source of this is phospholipid, a principle component of the cell membrane. Thus the conversion of arachidonic acid to prostaglandin may have something to do with regulating the membrane's functions. The cell membrane itself appears to be the prime site for the formation of prostaglandins that it produces as needed.

The interrelation of FAs and prostaglandins raises questions about diseases arising from dietary deficiencies. Prostaglandin synthesis may be lowered in EFA-deficiency, thereby causing some of the effects of this condition. David A van Dorp and his coworkers in the Netherlands, found that only those FAs that serve as precursors for the synthesis of prostaglandins can cure an EFA deficiency in rats. This suggests that some less obvious, perhaps metabolic, aspect of EFA deficiency is due, in part, to failure to synthesize necessary prostaglandins. The possible relevance of this to multiple sclerosis has recently been highlighted by a report that the synthesis of prostaglandins is markedly lower in multiple sclerotics than in controls.

In terms of the "bystander mechanism" model of multiple sclerosis, therapy theoretically should be directed towards suppression of the local immune reaction in the central nervous system. PUFAs, as substances able to enter freely in a blood-brain relationship, could be of great practical importance. But the potential benefit of long-term dietary linoleic acid supplements in multiple sclerosis must be regarded with the greatest caution pending the results of further careful investigation. No one can recommend the management of an "at risk" multiple sclerotic by PUFA, where it may well be justifiable to accept possible risks of treatment, unless these risks are fully appreciated.

Before turning to this matter, however, two points must be made. First, a statement of the fundamental principle of biologic dietetics: namely, that the food requirements of man are neither haphazard nor capricious. They are what they are for logical and intelligible reasons. In terms of the Darwinian concept of adaptation, "the optimum diet of man consists of those foods he has eaten in his evolutionary past."[105] Thus "optimum" foods for man are those concatenations of chemicals he has eaten in evolutionary time and during the evolutionary process. They are assemblages of chemicals wherein the quantity of different elements and compounds varies from a trace (some recent work suggests the need for small amounts of silicon, tin and vanadium) to preponderant amounts and percentages.

In essence, an optimum diet means eating these chemical clusters. They contain the dietary components to which man has adapted and which have supported his evolution. And these components would be best utilised in the context of their natural occurrence. No other feeding should be considered wholly correct and any other feeding should be suspect. For example, large doses of vitamin C may reduce the incidence of the common cold, but they may also have some secondary effect as yet not envisaged or detected. Similarly, sugar ingested separately from its dietary context is not a food as herein defined.

Corollary to the idea of adaptation is that of maladaptation to the eating of anything but "optimum" foods. The degree of maladaptation is the measure of the degree of malnutrition. And even if the generally accepted minimum requirements of all known food elements are in the diet, the simultaneous intake of large additional quantities of one or more dietary components may effectively produce malnutrition. Moreover, we must give adequate consideration to the perspective of time in nutrition. Even marginal dietary deficiencies and imbalances must produce cumulative effects neither looked for nor recognised when they appear. Long-term dietary abuse is bound to eventuate in small daily effects which are additive, and culminate in an observable pathology.

The second point is that advice to laymen on medical matters calls for a fine sense of judgment. On occasion, recommendations can be made with certainty because the scientific evidence is unequivocal. Such occasions are rare generally, and certainly nonexistent with regard to the therapeutic use of PUFAs in multiple sclerosis. Statements which urge or even support dietary supplementation with them lack judgment on the crucial issues of effectiveness and safety.

Interest in PUFA was aroused initially by a postulated etiologic link between saturated fats and heart disease. The lipid-lowering effect of PUFAs in humans has been known for twenty years, and the consumption of vegetable oils for this purpose became widespread in Scandinavian and North American countries about ten years ago. The Boards of Health in the former recommended major dietary changes involving the substitution of PUFA for saturated fatty acids to the general public. In the United States, the advice offered by authoritative bodies such as the American Heart Association, the Food and Nutrition Board of the National Academy of Science, and the Council on Foods and Nutrition of the American Medical Association has strongly favoured dietary change. Statements such as "the evidence now available is sufficient to warrant taking prudent action (dietary change) at this time in the population at large" came from these organisations as recently as 1973.[106]

In keeping with this trend, scientists in Australia have developed feed supplements for the production of polyunsaturated ruminant meat and milk fat. These consist of vegetable oils embedded in a matrix of treated protein from the oil seed and from added casein. The linoleic acid of the feed supplements is effectively protected from ruminal hydrogenation and is readily incorporated into milk fat and adipose tissue. An Australian research institute has entered into a licence agreement for the development and commercial production of polyunsaturated meat and milk products with Dalgety Agri Lines Pty. Ltd., a company formed for the purpose by the United Kingdom and United States controlled parent companies.

Western communities, however, have been exposed to PUFAs for a relatively short time and even if the immunosuppressive effects of EFAs were not suspected it would be reasonable to suppose that long-term dietary supplementation/substitution could have harmful effects. One diet-heart trial substituting PUFAs for saturated fats conducted in Los Angeles in 1972 indicates an increased incidence of cancer in groups using PUFAs. One reason may be the lengthy exposure of the group to the PUFA diet; the initiation and establishment of cancer takes time. Secondly, the participants were elderly, so they may have had an extended or peculiar exposure to carcinogens. Perhaps the PUFA diet promoted cancer previously initiated, and was not itself a source of carcinogen.

In any event, we now know that PUFAs and cancer may be related. Fats can promote cancer in at least two ways. First, they may actually be carcinogenic; corn oil, rich in polyunsaturated triglyceride FAs, is in mice, for example. If the fat itself is carcinogenic, it will be impossible to reduce the carcinogenicity of PUFAs. However, it is more likely that most, if not all, of the carcinogenicity is due to the breakdown products of fats, or to contaminants from nonfat sources.

Autoxidation of PUFAs results in the formation of potentially carcinogenic lipid peroxides. Not only are they extremely toxic but they also bind strongly to gastric mucosal cells. The peroxide forming capacity of the fat is reduced if a suitable antioxidant is added. Vitamin E is a natural antioxidant.

Interestingly, Mickel has suggested that the fall in linoleic acid concentrations in multiple sclerotics might reflect a depletion by peroxidation processes.[55] Peroxidised PUFA would cause platelet aggregation in the post-capillary venules of the central nervous system, attacking the tissue directly and bringing about protein denaturation. Protein denatured in this way would become antigenic, prompting development of an autoimmune process responsible for the progress of the disease.

In support of this idea, peroxidized arachidonic acid has been shown *in vitro* to cause changes in platelet adhesiveness similar to those found in multiple sclerotics. Further, diets rich in PUFA and poor in natural or synthetic antioxidants are known to cause nutritional encephalomalacia (NE) in chicks. This is an acute disease of the nervous system following feeding of a diet deficient in vitamin E and enriched with linoleic acid, both necessary prerequisites for the development of NE. The antioxidant activity of the vitamins and the easy oxidizability of linoleic acid suggest the disease is somehow related to lipid peroxidation. The products of peroxidation have not been demonstrated in the brains of affected chickens examined immediately after death, but the development of acute neurologic signs and death has been reported in chickens given peroxides of linoleic acid. Injection of linoleyl hydroperoxide into chicks predisposed to NE by the appropriate diet, but not actually showing signs of the disease, causes considerable cerebellar damage and congestion of the capillaries of the brain.

Mickel's theory seems to contradict that of Dr. Swank, which proposes that a diet rich in animal fats (primarily saturated) increases the risk of multiple sclerosis. But PUFAs are more liable to peroxidation than saturated fats. Mickel, however, deals with this discrepancy by claiming that animal fat — as opposed to oil — contains a lower level of natural antioxidants. He suggests that increased PUFA peroxidation in multiple sclerosis may follow an enteric infection, possibly by a virus. Lysosomal enzymes released through enteric inflammation promote the peroxidation, and the inflammatory damage increases peroxide absorption from the gut, or alternatively, absorption of endotoxin, which stimulates peroxidase activity within the body. In other words, endotoxin producing infection is linked to central nervous system demyelination. However, an increase in lipid peroxides (or peroxidase activity) has not yet been demonstrated in multiple sclerosis. In fact, it may be impossible to do so as lipid peroxides need only be present in minute quantities.

Polycyclic hydrocarbons are toxic and potentially carcinogenic substances that can be produced by heating PUFAs. Benzpyrene has been detected in margarine and other vegetable fats, but not in butter. This suggests that ruminants act in some way as a benzpyrene filter. Margarine is a hydrogenated oil and, almost simultaneously with its spread throughout the states of North America in the fifties, the incidence of multiple sclerosis doubled. "Unfortunately, the type of damage is not due only to the use of hydrogenated oils, as a butter substitute, but also includes those hardened oils as components of a great variety of bakery products as well as some commercial ice creams and possibly even commercial salad dressings. The fact that margarine has now replaced butter by more than 50 percent suggests it may be a basic cause of multiple sclerosis development."[57] However, the amounts of polycyclic hydrocarbons present in vegetable fats can be reduced by active carbon treatment.

The most disturbing findings regarding the relationship between PUFAs and cancer concern the potentiation of the tumour-inducing properties of other carcinogens by unheated PUFAs. Very little has been done to elucidate their promoting or potentiating ability. Nevertheless, Drs. West and Redgrave speculate on the possible effects. In their opinion, these include the protection of the carcinogen from metabolic destruction or excretion; changing the membrane composition of cells to facilitate access of the carcinogen to its site of action (the rate of diffusion of some substances across model membranes is increased when the lecithins of membranes are highly unsaturated); changing the chromosomal stability; changing the DNA repair potential; influencing the immune response by a depression of phagocytosis or an induction of immune paralysis to particular antigens mediated through a change in cell receptor. (A "paralysed" lymphocyte is no longer capable of being stimulated. Paralysis can occur when a lymphocyte is confronted by very high concentrations of antigen; it can also result from the continuous presence of extremely small antigen concentrations, below the threshold required for stimulation. Paralysis leads to the immune system tolerating its own antigens, which can then proliferate.)

Vitamin E deficiency also appears to be linked with PUFAs. In premature infants receiving formula mixtures containing fat with a relatively high content of PUFAs, a syndrome comprising oedema, skin lesions and elevated platelet count and morphologic changes in erythrocytes has been described. The lesions and haematologic changes were associated with low plasma vitamin E levels and increased erythrocyte sensitivity to peroxide haemolysis. These abnormalities disappeared rapidly after the administration of vitamin E and were not observed in infants fed identical diets supplemented with vitamin E. Rats fed high linoleic acid-containing diets also have an increased need for vitamin E to prevent haemolysis. And it has been reported that rats fed diets deficient in vitamin E develop muscular dystrophy.

Increased plasma vitamin E concentrations and decreased red cell haemolysis were noted in a group fed a diet rich in PUFAs containing adequate vitamin E. This shows the necessity of proper supplementation of PUFA diets with vitamin E to reduce the possibility of adverse effects. Harris and Embree propose that "adequacy" of dietary vitamin E be defined as the presence of 0.6 mg per gram of PUF. Unfortunately, the requirement of vitamin E is not related in a simple way to PUF intake. Thus one study directed at the question showed no evidence of vitamin E deficiency in the serum of persons eating PUFA. According to these investigators, the ratio of vitamin E to linoleic acid in diets based on vegetable oils ought to be sufficient to counteract the oxidative effects of PUFA, since increasing the intake of vegetable oils will also raise the intake of vitamin E. For this reason, there has been general endorsement of safety and nutritional adequacy of diets in which PUFA partly replace other fats. But the finding in the Los Angeles study that there is a significantly increased incidence of gallstones in the group receiving the PUF diet has some theoretic basis; the solubility of cholesterol in bile might be disturbed by changes in cholesterol and bile acid excretion.

Other experiments suggest that rats fed on a diet rich in PUFs (corn oil) require more biotin and vitamin B_{12}. Vitamin B_{12} deficiency (evaluated by growth retardation) was produced by a PUF diet, but not by one containing beef tallow as the sole dietary fat. There do not appear to be any reports of increased requirements for B_{12} and biotin in humans fed diets rich in PUFs. However, in the light of the findings from animal studies, diets containing PUFs should contain at least the minimum requirements of these vitamins. Similarly, experiments with rats reveal an increased requirement for vitamin A in the presence of PUFs, due perhaps to the increased oxidative destruction of vitamin A. Since many PUF-rich vegetable oils have a low content of vitamin A, it is important that food preparations based on these products be supplemented.

The story of the gluten-free diet as a therapy has great human interest. Some years ago the feature writer of a reputable journal became interested in the fate of Roger MacDougall, a playwright well known in the immediate post-war period, who had vanished below the literary horizon. His probe revealed that the playwright, though still alive and well and living in London, had developed multiple sclerosis. After the brief therapeutic flirtation with neurology so devastatingly familiar to most multiple sclerotics, he turned to naturopathy, one of a variety of excursions which most of us also know so well. He chose a regimen based on the removal of gluten from the diet. In MacDougall's view it is this — a protein found in wheat, barley, rye and oats — in combination with dairy produce and refined sugar that is the root cause of the degenerative diseases, of which multiple sclerosis is one. "I had lost the proper use of my eyes, my hands, my legs, my voice; I was a helpless cripple," MacDougall writes.[59] However, he improved gradually, and about five years after beginning the diet found himself in good physical shape, active and with normal vision. (Interestingly, although MacDougall claims to be "as fit as any normal man of my age," some neurologic abnormalities can be detected on objective examination.)

The feature writer was so impressed by his find that his published article dealt less with MacDougall's literary achievements than the great benefits of the gluten-free diet to him. Thereupon a veritable avalanche of inquiries on the subject descended on almost every neurology department in Great Britain and the United States. Again the therapy seemed harmless enough and under the social pressures exerted, a small study was undertaken. The conclusion of Dr. Liversedge, a thoroughly down-to-earth writer on the disease, was that the diet is unlikely to influence favourably the *progress* of multiple sclerosis, and certainly does not affect the relapse rate.

Despite the small number of sufferers in his study, there seems to be no reason to quarrel with Dr. Liversedge's deduction; but neither is it apparent that MacDougall's famous claim that his remission is due to the diet he adopted, is ill-founded. It is a diet without gluten or refined sugar, low in saturated and rich in poly-unsaturated fats. Since the removal of gluten almost always results in depletion of the B group vitamins, of the utmost importance in neurologic disorders, the diet involves the intensive intake of these and others, as well as minerals. Nowhere does MacDougall claim that his diet is a *cure;* it is merely a possible means of facilitating, or at best not preventing the very poorly understood process of regeneration.

"You may ask," writes MacDougall, "why should I not get this treatment from a neurologist? The answer is simple. Multiple sclerosis is *not* a neurologic disease; the training undergone by a neurologist is not relevant to the problems of the condition. He may offer you drugs which may help in the short term. But multiple sclerosis is a condition . . ."

Multiple sclerosis, I think, is a syndrome rather than a condition or disease entity, with demyelination as only one of its signs, the extent of which (or even its presence) may vary from case to case. The reason for this variation is that multiple sclerosis is *not*, as MacDougall rightly insists, a neurologic disease, but a syndrome of ecologic origin. Those who benefit from a gluten-free diet probably do so because the allergenic substance responsible for the multiple sclerotic plaque has been removed. The failure to alter the relapse rate is due to the phenomenon of masking. Moreover, it is chemical contaminants, not the foods themselves, that are to blame. For example, gluten is contained in — among dozens of other substances — monosodium glutamate, a meaty-tasting flavouring agent which has recently come under fire in the *British Medical Journal* as causing the condition quaintly named Kwok's Quease, or the Chinese Restaurant Syndrome.

Dr. Robert Kwok, who practises in America, regularly eats Chinese food. One day, in a Chinese restaurant, he was suddenly seized with the most frightful gripping pain in his chest, running up into his neck. He felt that he was going to faint and more or less collapsed across the table. The acute pain, which he thought was the beginning of a heart attack, subsided after a few minutes, but it left him shaken and determined to find out what had instigated such alarming symptoms. After much research with interested colleagues, he eventually came up with the answer: he had an allergy to monosodium glutamate, which some Chinese chefs add in considerable quantities to the food they prepare. Kwok first published his own case in the *New England Journal of Medicine,*[45] and his name and the syndrome associated with it have since become well known to doctors throughout the world.

Every allergic person has her special target organ(s), areas of the body which tend to be involved in allergic reactions, often of the most obscure origin, time after time. In some this is an area of brain tissue and if it happens to be in that part responsible for muscular movement, the allergy may manifest as an epileptic seizure, or at least produce a metabolic encephalograph. Randolph has a film of a wheat-sensitive woman who had fits every time wheat was fed to her, while other foods, to which she was not allergic, had no such effect. If the part of the brain controls certain behavior patterns, then allergic irritation will produce recognisable mental or behavioral changes, changes that may be repeated whenever one particular allergen is applied to a particular person.

The problem is that man's metabolism, like all his self-regulatory processes, is genetically linked to eons past. The move from vegetarian tree dwelling to carnivorous ground hunting was achieved only with serious hardship and a high death rate. These changes took place a million or more years ago. One obvious visible addition was the sharp canine teeth which are useful for meat eating. Infinitely more important was the evolution of new metabolic pathways within the cells of the body. These enabled the liver and other tissues to convert animal fats and proteins (instead of the old vegetable foods) into substances to supply energy to the muscles and other organs. These new pathways allowed our hominid ancestors to utilise chemical building blocks, mainly unsaturated fats supplied by the flesh of herbivores, for growing the bigger and supposedly better brain that is the pride and downfall of contemporary man.

The complicated chemical reactions at cell level are dependent on a host of enzymes (physiologic catalysts) that have been perfected through thousands of generations living on natural foods, first wild plants and roots and later free-running fat meat. When we suddenly confront our finely adjusted body chemistry with huge dollops of refined starch, sugar and a host of brand new, synthetic chemicals, we literally guarantee a breakdown in our basic cell processes.

It is not easy to appreciate how enormously perilous it is to tamper with our enzyme systems. In 1959 Dr. Vogel introduced the term *pharmacogenetics* into clinical medicine. This is the study of genetically determined variations that are revealed *solely* by the effects of drugs. The genetic variation results in the absence or insufficiency of certain enzyme systems. The classical example of a pharmacogenetic disease is the hemolytic anaemia suffered by some members of certain ethnic groups, specifically, Mediterranean basin dwellers and Negroes. Brisk hemolysis may follow exposure to many common therapeutic agents, such as phenacetin, and even the fava bean apparently provokes the anaemia on the same basis. The cause is a genetically transmitted defect that results in a deficiency of a certain enzyme. Sufferers are perfectly normal clinically; they have no morphologic or physiologic abnormality of their red cells *until* one of the provocative drugs is given. Then brisk hemolysis occurs. Hemoglobin Zurich is another example; if a Swiss family had not been given sulfonamide drugs it is probable that this disease would have continued to escape detection.

In view of the multitude of known enzyme systems, as well as those suspected but not yet identified, many reactions to the chemical environment will soon be gathered into the fold of pharmacogenetic disorders or acquired enzyme insufficiencies.

However, as the introduction of new enzymes is probably continuous, no doubt we will eventually develop the ability to digest gluten, and myriad other exotics, harmlessly; unfortunately, that does not help those of us who are suffering now. A partial answer, perhaps, is for biochemists to develop artificial enzymes as an alternative to a diet free of indicated allergens. But, then, intolerance to wheat is not necessarily due to its gluten content. Wheat is the highest in gluten as well as one of the leading cereal grains demonstrated to be associated with food allergy. The pragmatic fact is that where there is clinical intolerance to wheat or to anything else, total abstinence is the best treatment.

The only way to keep our metabolism as it is presently constituted in good working order, is to take into account the roles in nutrition of foods *vis à vis* their biologic origins and interrelationships. And, moreover, to recognise particularly that the impact of foods is accentuated by individual susceptibility to specific examples, or by deficiencies in the ability of certain persons to metabolise given foods. In contrast to analytic dietetics the interest here is on food in the form actually ingested.

More specifically, this means food in the sense of its biologic identity, such as wheat, corn and other closely related cereal grains; with milk and the closely related beef; or with tomato and potato, red and green pepper, and tobacco — all members of the same biologic family. Individual susceptibility not only commonly exists to such biologically identified whole foods or their refined products, but also readily spreads to biologically related dietary items.

A biologic dietetics is also concerned with chemical additives and contaminants of given foods, as well as with the cumulative intake of these in both food and water supplies. Protein food, for example, may be contaminated chemically by feeding livestock with forage or grain containing insecticide or weed killer chemical residues; spraying or dipping animals for insect control; employing antibiotics and synthetic hormones as growth stimulants; washing dressed carcasses with detergents; dipping dressed fowl or fish in antibiotic solutions as a preservative and wrapping these foods in odorous wrapping materials. Many of these chemical contaminants are apparently concentrated in the fat of the meat.

This is interesting in view of the proposed etiologic connection between diets high in saturated fats and multiple sclerosis, despite the fact that modern man's body chemistry is presumably meat-adjusted. Moreover, the incidence of the disease among white South Africans, whose diet in this respect is hardly ideal, has only recently begun to increase. The question then, is whether saturated fat *per se* is the offender.

In few developed countries is farming still controlled by simple country folk, and meat free running. The first animal to be removed from the natural conditions of the traditional farm and subjected to intensive farming methods was the chicken. The essential step in turning it from a farmyard bird into a manufactured item was confining it indoors. This means that, among the many other vices of agribusiness, it does not breathe air that is not heavy with ammonia from the chicken's own droppings.

Today intensive farming is practised primarily in respect of pigs, cows, lambs and turkeys. The dual aims of veal production, for example, are to produce a calf of the greatest weight, and to keep its meat as light-coloured as possible. To achieve the first, the calf must take in a maximum amount of food; consequently, it is given no water. The calves' only source of liquid is their food — a rich milk replacer (the calf is separated from its mother) based on powdered milk and added fat. Light-coloured meat means keeping feeds deliberately low in iron. The calves develop a craving for it, and will lick any iron fittings in their stalls. In this they have been thwarted by confinement in wooden stalls. The anaemic calves lick the slats which become impregnated with their own urine, containing a modicum of iron despite a diet depleted of it. It seems highly unlikely that the rising incidence of multiple sclerosis in developing countries has anything much to do with implicated viruses being hastily transported by jumbo jet from the northern to the southern hemisphere, a suggestion made by more than one investigator.

Foods may also be contaminated by fumigants, fungicides, sulphur in various forms, artificial colouring, sweetening and ripening agents, protective waxes and impregnated containers, or by being cooked in chemically impregnated water. Foods canned in lined tins are contaminated by the phenolic resins used in the manufacture of some can linings.

Lead is one of a list of metallic elements capable of poisoning human beings. Chronic lead poisoning affects the nervous system, including the brain. Ankle drop, paralysis of the extremities and neurasthenia are prominent symptoms. At least three researchers have implicated lead as an etiologic factor in multiple sclerosis.[72] The *Consumer Bulletin* lists many foods and beverages with a high lead content, some no doubt because of lead arsenate insecticides, others because of lead parts in processing equipment.[17] Those especially high in the metal include baking powder, lobster claw meat, anchovy fillets, canned sardines, dried gelatin, whole wheat flour, puffed rice, quick-cooking oats, frozen corn, cola drinks, apple cider (commercial nonorganic) and vinegar, red wine and canned beer. Lead water pipes, lead paints, fumes from leaded gasoline and its exhaust products (which also enter foods), and glazed earthenware dishes can all add to our lead intake.

In an earlier issue of the same bulletin, the incidence of lead and arsenic in smoking tobacco was reported; tests of pipe tobacco revealed concentrations of lead up to eighty-five parts per million of lead. It was suggested that cigarette smoke may carry more lead to the lungs than pipe smoke does. The *British Medical Journal* noted that multiple sclerotics who resume smoking after a break in the habit "will experience worsening of ataxia, parethesiae and spasticity."[9]

Individuals adapt, or maladapt, to the cumulative ingestion of given excitants. This may be a food and/or those closely related biologically. It may involve the ingestion of a given chemical additive or contaminant or various closely related chemical additives and contaminants. The speed with which the adaptation-maladaptation process occurs and the relative severity of the resulting symptoms is proportionate to the degree of individual susceptibility involved. Under these circumstances, multiple cumulative environmental exposures to which different degrees of individual susceptibility and maladaptation exist conjointly assault a person at any one time.

Clinical reactions to the cumulative use of common foods were not recognised until the present century. Hare and, later, Brown pointed out the role of carbohydrates, especially cereal grains and sugars on the one hand, and protein foods, especially beef and milk on the other, in the etiology of migraine headaches. Benefits were reported as a result of diets avoiding these food groups and infractions of such diets were said to be associated with recurrences of headaches.

There is no such thing as a universally safe food. The singling out of certain foods as health foods, the categorising of organic foods as healthful and of nonorganic foods as noxious, the recommendation of unrefined foods as curative and refined foods as debilitating: all of these fashionable concepts are simplistic and misleading. To a given individual, any food in any of these pidgeon holes may be severely damaging. The lethal characteristics of milk may exercise vessication on some people. In such cases it is mistakenly used in a bland diet and may exacerbate an ulcerous condition. Honey is widely regarded as a safe sweetening agent. This ignores the fact that it contains bee allergens, allergens from specific plant nectars and allergenic polymers derived from sugars.

Establishing the existence of food allergy is exacting, difficult, time-consuming and individualised. Genuinely comprehensive environmental control is possible only in an ecologic unit under expert supervision; this is the *sine qua non* for the specific diagnosis of ecologic disturbances. The technique is especially effective in those manifesting multiple and/or advanced syndromes; those who have been on maintenance dosage of drugs, and particularly those susceptible and maladapting to a wide range of environmental exposures.

According to veteran Dr. Randolph, nutrition and dietetics is presently monopolised by a relatively narrow and essentially one-sided point of view, encapsulating a fundamental error in fact-gathering. This error, inherent in the analytic approach, imparts a static orientation to one of nature's most dynamic biologic relationships. There is nothing static about the fact that the clinical responses of the same person at different times are usually dissimilar. All diagnostic testing procedures must focus on the dynamic interrelationship between a given person and the ingestion of a specific foodstuff under precisely controlled circumstances.

MULTIPLE SCLEROSIS IS
A FAMILY AFFAIR

U NLESS the symptoms are severe, when the basic needs of the multiple sclerotic have to be met, little can be done *for* her. In an acute phase, however, if the family, or others, are to provide genuine caring, they need to understand their own feelings and reactions to the symptoms of the illness. Their often devastating emotional problems tend to be overlooked, or cast aside, because the multiple sclerotic is thought to be the only one suffering; and they experience considerable guilt when they give vent to pent-up feelings.

The sufferer may be the principal wage earner of the family, or a dependent young adult at home or in school. The affected family members could include spouse, children and parents. The family may comprise just the immediate household or an extended group with grandparents and other relatives. During the crisis of relapse the family is expected to cope with frustration, anger and anxiety; with hopelessness, helplessness and loss, while yet retaining its stability. The sufferer's inexplicable mood changes which are neither voluntary nor purely psychological, the often rapidly changing symptoms and levels of functioning, make adjustment difficult. Any kind of normal existence seems impossible.

A family that too quickly takes over and handles everything for the sufferer encourages not only dependency, but the development of secondary gains, the enjoyment of which dissuade the multiple sclerotic from continuing even at the level that is physically and mentally possible. Furthermore, premature intervention distorts the roles of family members that can have serious consequences for the children, impose strains that tear a marriage apart, and damage parent-child relations where the sufferer is still the child in an older family.

Realistic planning takes into consideration the physical needs of the individual and the kinds of care necessary to sustain the best possible functioning. In addition, members of the family can undertake an activity previously carried out by the ill member, when she is clearly unable to act in that capacity any longer. In more severe situations, assistance may extend to an increase in domestic help or a job for the wife, in order to replace the lost income of an ill husband.

Any of these measure must be weighed against the needs of *all* the members of the family. If income is a problem, for example, and a wife has to consider returning to work, the care of the young children must be so arranged that their development is not endangered. However, it is important for the spouse, and the marital and family relationships, that the individuals involved maintain their outside interests so as to enhance their integrity and self-esteem.

Wherever possible, the problems arising from the illness that relate to work, recreation and child care, etc., should be carefully discussed by all members of the family, *particularly the sufferer,* to establish an open and congenial atmosphere wherein planning and criticism of previous tactics is possible and, if necessary, corrected. Such planning and review must rest on a realistic appraisal of the sufferer's capacity for self-help. Wherever possible, she should be encouraged to continue those activities that are pleasing and productive. Where special aids and assistance are necessary to do this, the general practitioner can help with the planning.

Experienced general practitioners quickly learn that the multiple sclerotic, her family and friends need a great many hours of care and counselling, of realistic support and reassurance. The disease can result in physical disability of infinite variety. The doctor and family together combine knowledge and ingenuity to help the sufferer retain as much independence as possible when one or more parts of her body refuse to function properly. Canes, braces, slings, wheelchairs, commodes, chair lifts and many combinations of safety devices are now available to reinforce the greatest effort on her part to continue to be active.

In the exercise of choices and the development of adaptive

processes for dealing with the changing symptoms of the disease, there will be many emotional and psychologic reactions that are difficult to cope with. The moods and responses of the sufferer may at times be quite different from those to which the family has become accustomed. The marital relationship, or parent-child relationships, will be strained at those times. In the face of this unusual behavior, members of the family may doubt the appropriateness of their plans, or feel that the ill member no longer has the same feelings of love and concern for them.

Perhaps the most important help, for any family faced with multiple sclerosis, is the reassurance that they are not alone. Also the capricious nature of the disease process makes every multiple sclerotic family vulnerable and therefore less able than usual to manage effectively. Staying together, growing and developing despite the burden of multiple sclerosis is indeed a challenge to any family.

Home Nursing Skills: The Acute Phase*

The attitudes, interests and concerns of the family have a direct bearing on the multiple sclerotic's response to her new state. Patience and kindness, understanding and tolerance help her feel she is accepted as a person. Respect for age, recognition of her achievements, praise for her successes — all are important contributions to a possible remission.

Many activities that a healthy person does automatically — moving in bed, sitting, standing, walking — are, in fact, complex physical movements resulting from coordination between brain and muscle. When these are ingrained in us as habits, we forget completely that each step had to be learned and, in the case of the multiple sclerotic, may have to be relearned.

The way each person views her own handicap is largely a question of her emotional response to it. How eager, anxious or resistant she is toward her rehabilitation depends on what

*In addition to my own experiences, I have referred to the MS Home Care Program produced by the National Multiple Sclerosis Society, New York, in conjunction with American Red Cross, as well as to other books listed in further reading.

hope she has of learning to use her remaining capabilities. Ideally, she makes headway gradually from one stage to another, eventually becoming able to take care of herself independently of others. Some want to do things for themselves sooner than others. Some are unwilling to attempt anything until coaxed again and again to do so. And it is only realistic to recognise that there are those few who will never regain the ability to care for themselves.

In this chapter and the two that follow, a few selected skills as well as simple aids and devices are suggested to ease the burden of the home nurse, family member or friend and the disabled multiple sclerotic. An entire book could be devoted to this subject, but with a little thought and ingenuity these ideas can be used to develop a personal stock of tools, concrete and otherwise, that are most appropriate to the unique needs of the sufferer, her family and her friends.

The following are the basic principles of *home care*:

- Recognise how much the individual is capable of doing for herself.
- Never do more for her than is absolutely necessary, even if it does take less time for you to do it than to allow her to do it herself.
- Plan your time, and that of your charge, so that neither feels hurried or frustrated because something is taking longer than expected.
- Give the individual enough time to do whatever she can by herself. Whether washing her face or drinking from a cup, it has meaning in that she is still able to do something, to achieve at some level, no matter how minor it seems to you.
- No matter what you do, *avoid fatiguing* the individual.
- Always try to keep the disruption of personal and social routines to an absolute minimum. Attractive hairstyles or an intimate meal with a friend(s) are not impossible simply because the individual is bed-bound.
- Each activity comprises many individual steps and the inability to do any one of these will prevent the person from eventually accomplishing the activity independently.

- Use adapted equipment whenever necessary to enable the person to accomplish an activity independently.

These are the basic principles in respect of *aids and devices*:
- Individual approaches to home care, activities of daily living, homemaking or dressing, depend entirely upon the extent and severity of the handicap, or on the "tricks" that can be utilised. A technique may be devised to overcome a particular problem, making aids and devices or more drastic modifications unnecessary. Alternatively, techniques and manoeuvers can be used in conjunction with aids.
- Do not buy costly aids until their need and worth have been proved. Large expenditure is justified only if the aids can be operated successfully and do their job over a long period of time. When aids are recommended as a temporary measure until full or partial recovery of function, they should be inexpensive or, preferably, improvised at home.
- If, like many multiple sclerotics, you are, in effect, one-handed:
  Either fix your work, *or* the tool you use.
- Use light-weight implements, e.g. plastic knives and forks.
- If your grip is very weak, either pad the handle of your implement with foam rubber or attach a strap or piece of shaped plastic that fits over your hand.
- Improvise methods for lengthening handles, e.g. toothbrushes, knives. Provide a gutter for the thumb.
- Keep equipment simple and take thought in deciding what you really need. Do not fill your home with gadgets and gimmicks you may use only once.

During an acute phase of the illness, the multiple sclerotic may be relatively helpless, requiring attention to her basic needs in bed. A comfortable position in bed is partially achieved through support for the spinal curves with a pillow under the head and neck, or a flat pad in the small of the back. A smooth, firm but resilient mattress is also necessary.

Sick people tend to curl up in bed with the back, hips and

knees flexed. This could be to ease pain or keep warm, but if the multiple sclerotic stays like this for long, it becomes increasingly difficult for her to regain correct body position. Also, changing position frequently promotes circulation and relieves prolonged pressure on any one part of the body. It is a mistaken kindness to permit someone who does not want to be disturbed to remain static for any length of time. In hospital nursing, two hours is considered the maximum time to lie in one position.

Deterioration is fairly rapid in joints and muscles. Normally, the flexor (bending) muscles and the extensor (straightening) muscles are in balance. Sometimes this is affected, and one type of muscle is shortened. To prevent these *contractures,* adequate support must be given to weakened muscles. Generally, the weaker ones are those that extend or turn outward or upward. The stronger muscles bend or turn inward. Bending your finger requires stronger muscles than straightening it. This applies equally to muscles in the foot; support must be given to the feet to prevent "foot drop," to the paralysed hand to prevent claw-like deformity and to the outer parts of the thighs to prevent hip deformities.

Another threat to the bed-bound is *pressure sores* (decubitus ulcers). The combination of pressure from prolonged periods in the same position, associated with immobility and/or sensory deprivation, plus friction on the skin created by involuntary spastic movements, or being dragged across bed linen, leads to this complication. Most often, these ulcers occur over the bony prominences of the body, that is, the base of the spine, shoulder blades, elbows, heels and even ears can be sites of pressure.

Pressure, too, is avoided by regular change in position. In less severe bedridden stages, the multiple sclerotic can help to turn herself. In more severe stages, the moving must be done for her. Support the joints when moving extremities to prevent strain or deformity. The extremities are positioned so that they remain in correct body alignment.

Certain protective aids may prevent ulcers. At times, an inflatable rubber ring produces the desired effect. A more elaborate aid is the flotation pad, a square of silicone material placed under areas of greatest pressure in bed or in a chair to minimise the degree of pressure on the skin. Sheepskins, if kept clean and dry, aid significantly in skin care. In cases with markedly fragile skin and multiple areas of breakdown it may be necessary to resort to an alternating air pressure mattress or a water bed.

On awakening, the multiple sclerotic requires toilet care. The helpless person needs to have these services performed for her. The more able are encouraged to do as much as they can for themselves. The multiple sclerotic is offered a bedpan or assisted to the lavoratory. Hands and face are washed and teeth brushed in bed or bathroom.

The cap on the tube of toothpaste can be opened by holding it between the teeth. When closing the tube, place it into the cap and tighten. Special devices to which the handle of the brush is attached may be improvised or bought. For example, a nail file fixed in a wooden handle can be removed and the toothbrush handle inserted.

Care of dentures is possible if added precautions are taken to prevent their falling. Washing them in a basin might be a safe method.

Wherever possible the individual is encouraged to bathe herself. This provides exercise, stimulates circulation and gives the person that all-important sense of achievement and self-reliance. Only the acutely ill or helpless multiple sclerotic ought to be bathed by someone else.

Have the person move to the near side of the bed for convenience and ease in working. Remove her nightdress. As each part is bathed — neck, arms, shoulders, back, legs — place a towel beneath it to prevent bedding from getting wet and the person from getting chilled. Avoid dragging a wet face cloth; wring it out well and fold corners. Use long firm strokes when washing; use very little soap on the body, none on the face. Change water when soapy or cool. Wash, rinse and dry one part before moving on to the next. If skin is dry, body lotion is soothing.

Daily brushing and combing to keep her hair in a healthy condition can be accomplished by the multiple sclerotic through the use of special devices, such as long-handled combs

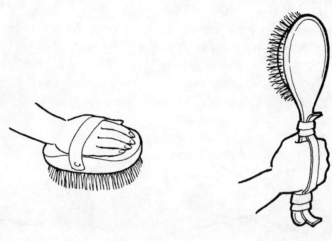

Figure 4.   Figure 5.

or brushes with special grips that attach to the hand. A tail comb can be set into a piece of wood.

For many women, hair care also involves perming. Ask your hairdresser to come to your home; if you are unable to set your own hair, she may also be prepared to make weekly visits, as mine was. However, you may enjoy making the effort to set your own hair.

Care of nails can be a problem. Anyone who uses an emery board may find it helpful to run nails over a sheet of fine sandpaper. Others prefer to use a nail clipper that has been

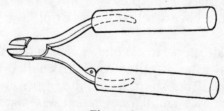

Figure 6.

fastened to large wooden handles or mounted in a paper stapling machine.

This integrated cosmetic tray, useful for the bed-bound as

well as those in wheelchairs, combines nail clippers, cream jars "held" in the tray, and an improvised emery board whose swinging action simplifies its use for both hands. There is absolutely no excuse for not being well-groomed!

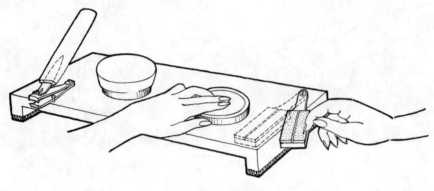

Figure 7.

With limitation of movement, stiffness of joints or poor coordination, self-care in respect of elimination is more difficult. Larger quantities of toilet paper are needed. For complete care it may be necessary to use a washcloth and towel. Dispensable towlettes are also available; to avoid clogging the plumbing, dispose of these in a paper bag.

Each bedpan episode can be a distressing experience for the helpless multiple sclerotic. Ordinarily the home nurse should not attempt to place a completely helpless person on a bedpan alone; she should have a helper to work opposite her across the bed.

Turn the multiple sclerotic on her side and steady her in that position. Place a large pillow or two small ones lengthwise against her back, from shoulders to the upper buttocks. Place a large pillow or two small ones lengthwise against her, from thighs to feet, building a platform. Protect the ends of the pillows and the bed between them with a waterproof sheet. Place the pan on edge against the buttocks, as exactly in the desired position as possible, hold it in place, and roll the multiple sclerotic back onto the pan and the platform of pillows.

Allow sufficient time for use of the bedpan. Hold it firmly on the bed while the helper rolls the multiple sclerotic towards her, onto her side, off the platform. Remove the bedpan and then the pillows. Cleanse, wash and dry the person. Turn her onto her back or position her comfortably on her side. Provide the necessary supports for proper body posture.

Some multiple sclerotics may lose control of their bladder and/or bowels, a condition known as *incontinence*. It creates a difficult situation for both the sufferer and home nurse. By the very nature of the disease, accompanying urinary symptoms are diverse. Urgency, increased frequency and precipitancy may occur, lasting perhaps a few weeks, or months or years. In some, acute retention of urine may be an initial problem, as the sensation of the bladder being full is impaired. The raised pressure in the distended bladder may force small amounts of urine out at intervals, causing dribbling. Loss of tone in the sphincter muscles may also lead to lack of control.

Protection of the bed and linens by flannel covered rubber or plastic sheets helps to reduce the time and energy expended on changing and laundering bedding. Sanitary pads may afford sufficient protection to women where there is only minor leakage, especially if worn with protective sani-briefs; a pad which "gels" when wet, and also contains a deodorant, gives particularly good protection. Where leakage is greater, Kanga Pants™ are comfortable to wear.

Because the skin comes in contact with bowel and urinary discharges, cleanliness and dryness are essential. Changing the multiple sclerotic and washing and drying the lower portion of the back should be done immediately. A special ointment or lotion may be necessary.

Deodorising powders, sprays, wicks, etc., are helpful in controlling odours. It has been found that a six-ounce glass of cranberry juice taken daily helps to control the unpleasant urine odours which the multiple sclerotic finds so upsetting.

If retention occurs, a little pressure with the fingers on the bladder can sometimes cause urination to begin. In the case of urinary incontinence a great deal can be done to improve some conditions by strengthening the pelvic muscles, using simple techniques carried out by the individual. Since improvement is gradual, patience and perseverance are essential.

1. Sit, stand or lie comfortably, without tensing the muscles of the seat, abdomen or legs; pretend you are trying to control diarrhea by tightening the ring of muscle around the anal sphincter. Do this several times until you feel certain that you have identified the area and are making the correct movement.

2. Sit on the lavatory or bedpan and commence to pass water; while doing so attempt to stop the flow in mid-stream by contracting the muscles round the front passage. Do this several times until you feel sure of the movement, and of the sensation of applying conscious control.

3. Exercise as follows: sitting, standing or lying, tighten first the muscles of the anal sphincter, then the front, and then both together. Count 4 slowly, and release the muscles. Do this four times, repeating the whole sequence once every hour. With practice the movements should be quite easy to master and the exercises can be done at any time.

Remember to repeat them daily for at least two to three months, as frequently as possible.

Bowel and bladder training establish a pattern of relatively systematic functioning which helps the multiple sclerotic and reduces the danger of infection. Since the multiple sclerotic is unable to feel when her bladder is full, she must learn other signs and symptoms: sweating and headaches may be indicative of its distension.

A simple bladder drill can be practised to diminish frequency. Whenever passing urine, stop the flow deliberately and then start it again; this is a method of control that can be recognised and made use of. Then try, by "holding on" in this way, to wait a little longer before passing urine the next time; this interval should gradually be lengthened, step by step, day by day. It takes time and patience to train the bladder, but, for example, hourly use of the bedpan can be extended to two-hourly use. This positive and practical action that the individual can take herself is of great value, especially when anxiety is a factor in frequency.

The amount and kind of fluid and food intake, the timing of eating and drinking and the regularity of attempts to void all influence the success of training. One way to cope with urinary incontinence is to ensure that the bladder is completely emptied. This can be accomplished *only* by sitting up or standing, because the bladder opening must be directed downward for complete emptying; you must give gravity a chance to do its work! If the multiple sclerotic lies on a bedpan, the bladder is only partially emptied and dribbling results. Where persistent overflow incontinence cannot be checked, drainage of the bladder by catheter may be necessary, *but this is a medical decision.*

After the multiple sclerotic has been in bed for a long time, she may need assistance to get out of bed, get into a chair from her bed or to walk. As her condition improves she can increase her strength by pushing herself to a sitting position with her hands. With growing skill in moving without help, she should be given less and less physical support.

Different manoeuvres help the multiple sclerotic to move herself and also aid the home nurse in moving her. When you move yourself try to lead your movements by pointing your head and/or face in the desired direction. There is a grain of truth in the saying that your body can go where your head will go. When in a sitting position also try to use your heels or feet to push, but first bend your legs at the knee. By pushing with the heel of each bent leg in turn, you tend to raise your tail on that side, facilitating a forward creep. Unfortunately, your arms are not long enough for hoisting yourself about, especially when seated on a springy surface. To "lengthen" your arms, place a thick book (or block) under each palm (see p. 204). Now practice raising your buttocks off your bed or chair — a good muscle strengthening activity.

Once these arm and heel thrusts have been mastered separately, start pushing with the arm and leg on the same side to raise the buttock on that side; then progress to pushing on the books with both arms and your best heel to move back- and forwards. Remember to keep your knee bent and your arms beside your body; push on all three points simultaneously to move your buttocks; then reposition books, hands and heel.

By pushing on your hands and heel with them pointing in the direction in which you wish to go, you should be able to turn around to sit on the side of the bed. By placing one arm a little out to one side and keeping the other close beside you, sideways travel is possible.

Even if you do not have a handle and rope attachment on the ceiling, you can still help yourself to sit up from a lying-down position. First, raise your head, then pull on a rope ladder attached to the footrail of the bed, or to a stabilised chair in the absence of a footrail.

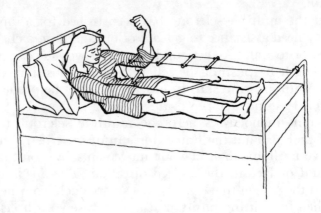

Figure 8.

Turning over can be difficult. From prone (facing down) push the toes of your stronger leg under the ankle of the other; using your hand bent up so that you push on the surface immediately under the shoulder you can now roll to either side. As you do this, lift your head up and towards the side to which you intend to roll.

To turn back again to prone put your weaker arm over your head, bend the leg on the side away from which you intend to turn, push on the floor at waist level with the hand on the same side, life up your head and look where you are going as you "thrust."

Rocking is a manoeuvre for getting out of a chair or off the bed onto your feet. Small rocking movements forward and back are started, each increasing in size by making a bigger effort at the appropriate moment, thereby adding to the power and size of the total movement. Sit towards the front edge of your chair or bed. Lean forwards so that your head is over your knees; pull your feet back so that they too are under your knees. Place your hands on your knees or chair arms. Start to push on your hands and feet and try to push your head forwards and upwards; drop back onto the chair. Repeat immediately so that as you bounce forwards after the drop back, you apply another push on your hands; your tail should rise further off the chair. Even if you cannot stand without help, this is an excellent exercise.

Activities of Daily Living (ADL)

ADL refers to all those day-to-day self-care activities that a healthy person takes for granted, but which being multiple sclerotic renders problematic and time consuming. There are, however, tricks and short-cuts for solving all kinds of problems, and many appliances, large and small, to make disability easier to cope with.

The basic principles of the *activities of daily living* are as follows:
- Recognise your potential capabilities.
- Each self-care activity comprises many individual steps and the inability to do any one of these will prevent you from accomplishing the activity independently.
- You need time to complete each activity without being rushed.
- You must do as much for yourself as possible.
- Only use adapted equipment when absolutely necessary.

All those activities that go into maintaining the family contribute to its stability and well-being. These are an assortment of special physical tasks and executive functions as well as the creation of an emotional atmosphere that help to hold the family together. Disruption of this complex routine tends to weaken the whole family. If this can be minimised, stability can be sustained; however, if it cannot, all those concerned may have to learn new roles.

It is here that the multiple sclerotic often has the greatest difficulties. Reconciling oneself to *any* limitation is never easy; the outrageous fortune of chronic disability can be overwhelming. But before the multiple sclerotic who is disabled, or merely handicapped, can reenter community life as an active member, she must first be able to fend for herself within her own home. Obviously some tasks are beyond her capacity, but friends and family will notice snags and offer their help as a matter of course. Equally, the multiple sclerotic should not let her pride keep her from seeking assistance where this is necessary and as often as necessary.

Mobility

The ability to remain mobile is essential even where this depends on aids. Wheelchair, ambulation with aids and independent ambulation are a natural progression from the viewpoint of relative self-sufficiency.

Initially, rejection of a wheelchair by a multiple sclerotic is often intransigent. She feels she is "not sufficiently disabled," or that to use such an aid is "lazy," or will in some way stop her walking. In fact, it is the very person who regards herself as "insufficiently disabled" who gets the best value out of a wheelchair, because she becomes skilled in its management in a good phase instead of during a relapse or intercurrent illness when the effort is so much greater. She will, unless very unfortunate in her employment and domestic architecture, find that she can do more with less effort and fatigue when using a wheelchair; it is much easier to carry the laundry or office files around this way than when walking with stick or crutch. Also she may once more find the time and energy for activities that had become too great a struggle. The chair need only be used intermittently. You do not have to sit in it day and night once it is delivered! Using it on appropriate occasions may reopen activities abandoned because of the walking distances involved.

The correct prescription of a self-propelled wheelchair is important. A variety of factors govern the selection of the right one. The most common model is the Universal™, with the larger wheels at the back. It can be used indoors and outdoors, promotes better posture, permits easier transfer activities — the movement from here to there — and can be tilted to go up curbs and stairs. The Traveller™ has the larger wheels in front. It is used only indoors or on level surfaces; promotes poorer posture; is more difficult for transfer; and cannot be used for curbs or stairs. Chairs powered by motor are invaluable for those with no means to propel themselves.

Individual needs are the primary consideration in choosing wheelchair accessories. These are valuable in accomplishing daily living activities and maintaining the comfort and proper body alignment of the multiple sclerotic. Accessories, which should be selected by someone able to analyse the individual's disabilities and potential ability, include brakes which are *not* standard equipment. However, every wheelchair must be equipped with brakes for safety. Five-inch front casters are standard equipment, but the eight-inch caster allows for better control of the wheelchair; i.e. turning, rolling over rough surfaces and manoeuvering in small spaces. In addition, there are armrests, backrests, legrests, footrests and seat cushions.

Techniques for using a wheelchair also vary according to individual needs. This is relatively straightforward where both arms are available, but pushing one wheel only automatically turns the chair in a circle. Push the wheel with the one good hand and at the same time use one good foot to pull the chair in opposition, thereby countering the turn and allowing the chair to go forward.

A transfer is a pattern of movements whereby the multiple sclerotic moves from one surface to another. A safe transfer depends on proper equipment, firm stable surfaces and correct technique; safety devices such as rubber pads under each leg of the bed and chairs prevent slipping. Ideally, all transfers are learned using some means of assistance (a transfer belt or a firm guiding grasp around the waist) until the individual feels confident enough to manage independently.

For a successful transfer the multiple sclerotic must be able to achieve a sitting position and to maintain balance as well as hip elevation. These exercises help strengthen the upper extremities.

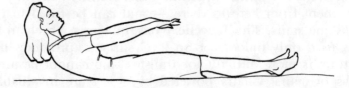

Figure 9.

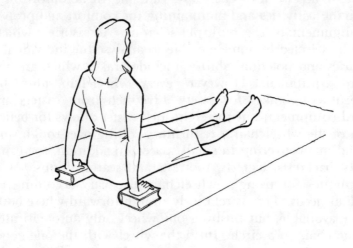

Figure 10.

The distance between the surface being transferred from and the item to which the person is transferring must be reduced to a minimum. Also allowances for differences in height between the two objects are necessary. The more techniques that are mastered and the more adjustments and changes in the placement of the wheelchair, bed or car that are possible, the easier transfer is in different situations.

Transfer from bed to wheelchair or vice versa is facilitated by a sliding board. This needs good sitting balance and arms powerful enough to raise hips off the bed. Another essential is a stable bed the same height as the seat of the wheelchair; a wheelchair with brakes, swinging detachable foot- and arm-rests, and a sliding board. The wheelchair with the *brakes locked* is placed next to the bed and facing towards its foot at a slight angle. The armrest on the side next to the bed is lifted up. When the multiple sclerotic is sitting upright the sliding board is placed between chair and bed.

To assume a sitting position, roll onto your side, place your legs — independently or with assistance — over the edge of the bed, and push your trunk to an upright position. Move closer to the edge, turning your knees away from the wheelchair and hips toward it. On turning adjust your feet with your hands to bring them directly under yourself. Lean over onto your *right* forearm, raising your left buttock off the bed; slide one end of the board beneath yourself. The other end must rest securely on the wheelchair seat. Using your upper extremities, move side-ways across the board onto the wheelchair. Lean over onto your *left* forearm and remove the sliding board.

Replace the armrest and swing the footrest into place. After placing your left foot on the footrest, unlock the brakes and move chair away from the bed. Finally, swing the right footrest into place and put your foot on it.

Eventually, with increase in upper extremity strength, transfer may be accomplished without the sliding board. You can practice "push-up" exercises to strengthen these muscles whenever you are in a sitting position. Place your hands on the bed next to your hips; straighten elbows, pushing on the bed and raising hips. Books or blocks under the hands "lengthen" your arms and improve the mechanics of the exercise. *Stop any exercise before fatigue level is reached.*

Independence in transferring to and from a toilet, and pri-vacy in its use, is important to all of us. Equalise the heights of the toilet and the wheelchair by installing a raised toilet seat, or a transfer bench that fits over the bowl and is the same height as the wheelchair. If accessibility of the toilet itself by the wheelchair poses a problem, use a commode chair as a substitute. You will also have to learn to adjust your clothing before and after transfer.

Position the wheelchair parallel or at an angle to the toilet. Lift your feet off the footrests, place them on the floor and swing footrests away. Move the chair until your knees are as close as possible to the toilet. *Lock Brakes.* Shift hips so that you are sitting sideways on the chair and move your legs so that knees are now away from the toilet.

Unlock brakes and move chair closer to the toilet. Relock brakes. While you still have the support of wheelchair armrests, loosen pants and by rocking from one side to the other, work them under buttocks.

Lift armrest. Place one hand on the opposite side of the toilet seat and the other on the wheelchair arm. Use your upper extremities to raise hips and move toward toilet. Several moves may be necessary to transfer. When accomplished, position lower extremities.

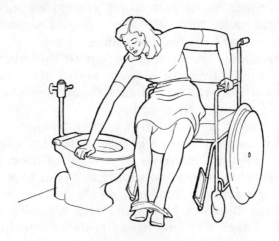

Figure 11.

In general, a shower is less strenuous than a bath since you can wash more easily seated on a stool in the shower. However, ensure that its legs have large suction-type grips.

If you prefer a bath, place wheelchair in a forward position as close as possible facing its side or end. *Lock Brakes.* Lift feet

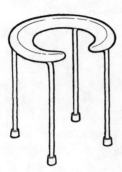

Figure 12.

and legs into bath. Placing hands on armrests of chair, slide body forward into a sitting position on edge of bath. Place one hand on the near edge of the bath and the other on the far side, or on safety grab-rail mounted on wall, and lower body into bath. Reverse procedure to return to chair.

It is easier to get in and out if the bath is filled with water, but be careful. To prevent slipping, use a rubber suction bath mat. If it is difficult to lower yourself into the bath place a small shower stool in the bath.

When moving in and out of bed and around the house is possible car transfers may be attempted. The principles are essentially the same though time may be important so that more proficiency at the outset is needed. Independent car transfers involve moving on the seat, opening and closing doors, and perhaps lifting the wheelchair in and out of the car.

Use the sliding board technique. Here a longer board — approximately 28″ to 34″ — is necessary to link the chair with the seat of the car. For those with strong muscles in the upper extremities and trunk, transfer without a sliding board.

Face the wheelchair toward the door of the car; open car door and swing it back to lock position. Move wheelchair forward into the angle formed by the car door and side of the car. *Lock brakes*. Slide to front edge of wheelchair seat and swivel around to face the wheelchair. Place hand nearest car door on the window ledge, and the other hand on the wheelchair armrest

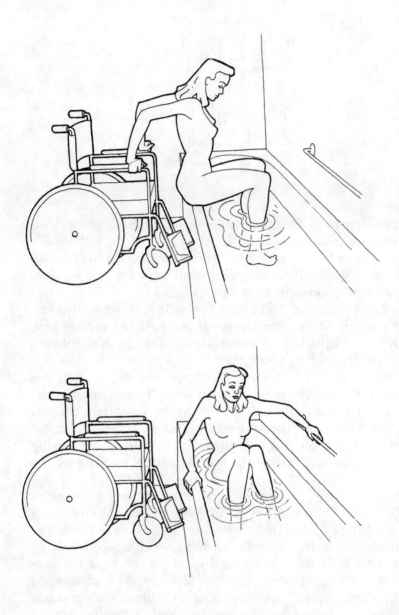

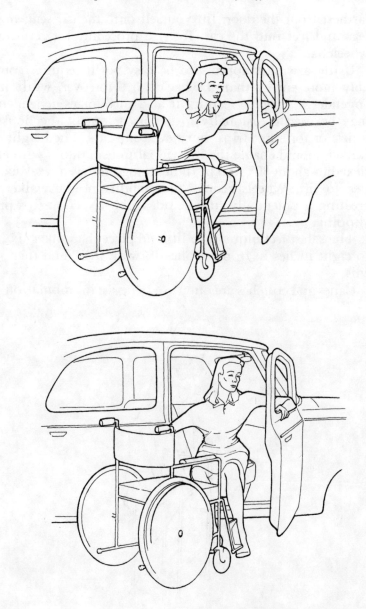

farthest from the door; lift yourself onto the car seat; now lift
legs and feet into the car. Reverse procedure for returning to
wheelchair.

Using a walker appears to be easy but it requires considerably more energy than a wheelchair. Moreover, while it does
engender a sense of security it also encourages dependence. It
may be used occasionally to get in or out of the house, the
toilet, or for short trips, but never on stairs. The height of the
walker should enable the individual to lean into it with elbows
flexed to about 30°, and be light enough for even weak extremities to lift. Wheels reduce the stability of the walker, thus
creating a potentially unsafe aid. Rubber suction tips prevent
slipping.

The safest technique is to lift and place the walker six inches
to eight inches in front of oneself, walk in it, and then repeat
this.

Canes and crutches are often used to assist in ambulation. They

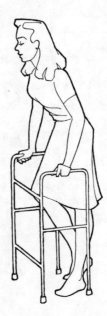

Figure 17.

call for the same physical capabilities as the walker, plus a more adept and secure balance. The axillary crutch fits under the upper arm, and the Lofstrand™ fits the forearm by means of a metal cuff which allows the individual to adjust clothes or grasp objects without losing the use of the crutch.

The type selected depends on the individual's physical condition, arm and trunk strength and/or body balance. The proper fit is essential and these aids should be used only with the approval and guidance of your general practitioner.

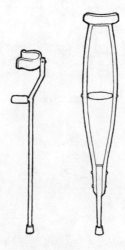

Figure 18.

Transferring from a wheelchair to crutches is not difficult. Place wheelchair, *brakes locked,* with back against the wall or a stable surface. Slide body to front edge of chair; place better leg back under the edge of the chair. Holding both crutches by the handpieces with one hand and placing the other hand on the armrest of the chair, push on hands, straightening the better leg, and bring body to standing position. Balancing on better leg and crutches transfer one crutch and then the other to underarm position. Reverse procedure to return to sitting position.

To master stairs with crutches, place one hand on bannister and both crutches under opposite arm; balance weight on hands

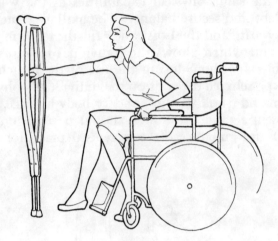

Figure 19.

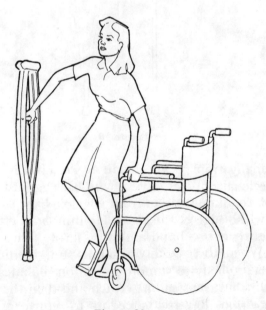

Figure 20.

and arms; step up with stronger leg; straighten stronger leg, thus lifting other leg and crutches. Continue up the stairs repeating the same pattern. Going down the stairs, move the crutches forward first, then the weaker leg, thus allowing the stronger leg to take the load of lowering the body weight.

A cane requires good control of the trunk and strength in arm and hand. The standard variety is available in different materials, such as aluminum or assorted woods. The four-legged cane has a ridged handgrip, legs which are narrowly juxtaposed, permitting its use on stairs, and it is usually made of aluminum. Safety suction tips prevent slipping.

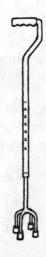

Figure 21.

Modification of the Home

One of the most disheartening experiences of a multiple sclerotic who, through effort and skill, achieves independence, is a home where it cannot be practised because of architectural barriers. When these are present, satisfactory adjustments or home alterations are necessary. There are various books on the subject of domestic planning that are included in the list of further readings. Too narrow doors and hallways, high windows with difficult latches, poor placement of electrical outlets, inaccessible cupboards, furniture arrangements with little manoeuvering space — all these are barriers to independence and create a hazardous home environment for the multiple sclerotic.

A few uncomplicated modifications to the home can increase the comfort and safety of those in wheelchairs. At least one outside entrance should be ramped or at ground level. The ramp must be a minimum of three feet wide with handrails thirty-two inches high, on at least one side. The surface of the ramp should be nonslip. Doors at least thirty-six inches wide open inward. Hallways less than four feet wide hinder wheelchair manoeuvers. No scatter rugs!

Lights and switches approximately three feet above the floor and horizontally aligned with door handles are convenient. Master switches in the living room, kitchen and bedroom are necessary. The wall telephone should not be more than four feet from the floor, with curtain pulleys and ventilating mechanisms also easily accessible.

Handrails on one or both sides of the toilet, twenty-six inches to thirty-three inches from the floor promote safety. A toilet seat of the correct height facilitates transfer. The bathroom must be able to accommodate a wheelchair comfortably. Mirror and medicine chest are so structured and situated that the person in a wheelchair can utilise them adequately. Accessories and alarm button are located about forty inches from the floor, and the bathroom door can be unlocked from either side.

The bath surface is anti-slip with a safety handrail securely mounted where it can be utilised for entrance or exit. A shower seat that is the appropriate height for transfer may be used if desired. All water controls must be within reach of a bathing position. Shower cubicles should be level with the ground, and the doorway at least thirty-two inches wide. A handrail on one side of the cubicle facilitates comings and goings. Handrails must be able to support 250 lbs., allow for three inches to four inches between bar and wall, be nonslip and devoid of sharp corners, with ends returning to the wall. A seat in the shower is essential, as are controls within reach, preferably a hand-held shower head.

In the bedroom a three-foot clearance for the wheelchair approach to the bed is the minimum possible. Outlets, switches and push-button alarm within easy reach of the bed are essen-

tial. Cupboards must provide sufficient storage space
with sliding doors and one rod no higher than forty-two
inches.

The kitchen is where many housewives choose to spend
much of their time, and if disability now deters them from
going out, they may seek compensation by extending their
homemaking activities. A well-planned kitchen is easier for
ablebodied and disabled alike. Many of the difficulties con-
fronting the latter can be overcome or mitigated by good planning and common sense. A well-planned kitchen can make the
time you spend there enjoyable and rewarding. In going about
this, consider the activities you and others will want to undertake there. It may be the most popular room in the house and
provide a comfortable centre for eating, hobbies, homework
and flower arranging. You may genuinely love to cook and
find relaxation in it; if so, remember special facilities for cake
or jam making.

As a general rule of thumb, all working surfaces should be
no higher than thirty-two inches to thirty-four inches. Open
areas beneath these provide space for a wheelchair. All storage
should be accessible and controls on equipment within easy
reach; dials should be large enough to read without straining
and contain safety devices. Doors on the refrigerator and oven
open sideways, or upwards, and again controls must be accessible, easy to read and equipped with safety devices.

You may feel at first that you need more adaptations and aids
in your kitchen than are, in fact, necessary and end up with
dozens of gadgets you never use. Keep your equipment simple
and take thought in deciding what you really need. Perhaps
practice with the equipment you have, plus rearrangement of
and minor modifications to your kitchen, are sufficient to ease
your burden to your own satisfaction. For example, it is an
obvious practical necessity to *fix your implement or piece of
equipment,* a bowl for instance, before starting to mix. One
way to do this is with "bowl holders," that is, holes the size of
your favourite bowls are made in a working surface or in a
pull-out work top.

Another way to fix an implement is by attaching a strap or

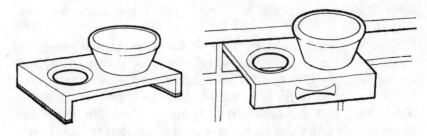

Figure 22.   Figure 23.

piece of shaped plastic to its handle that fits over your hand.

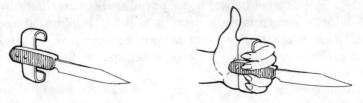

Figure 24.   Figure 25.

Most people seem to prefer to *secure* their *work*. The most useful aid is a chopping block with three or more thin vertical steel spikes on which a range of vegetables, fruit, meat, bread, etc., can be held in position for slicing. This is stabilised either by suction feet or by foam rubber stuck to the underside.

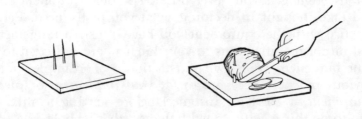

Figure 26.   Figure 27.

A vegetable holder with ten equally spaced sharp prongs about three inches long, set in either a stick or a hinged board, is a valuable aid. The holder, pushed into a vegetable or fruit, steadies it for cutting between the prongs — a neat way to slice cabbage, onions, beetroot or anything else. Success with tomatoes calls for a serrated knife.

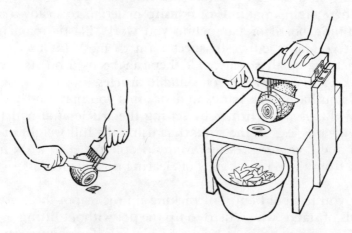

Figure 28.   Figure 29.

A spreading breadboard for one-handed people has been designed — a plain wooden board with beading along two sides against which the bread is pushed. A spike board is a useful alternative. One-handed people can spread as they would peel a potato, pulling the knife towards the thumb.

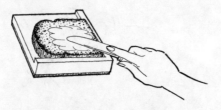

Figure 30.

Apart from fixing work, efficiency and comfort can be improved for most people, if they can steady what they are doing without keeping a tight hold on it. This applies particularly to those who have weak grip, are unsure or shaky, or tire easily. It is likely that fatigue will accentuate your symptoms, which can be frightening as you may assume that your condition is deteriorating. This is not, of course, necessarily so; you may just be overtired and will notice an improvement in yourself after a good rest, although possibly not immediately.

There are many kinds of nonslip materials to steady a bowl, chopping board or pan while you work. Plastic foam is the most common, either in sheet form or mesh (as used under carpets); a small square of either can be used on its own or stuck to the undersides of suitable articles.

If you have weak hands and/or arms you may find you can hold things more firmly by setting the article at arms length, downwards, e.g. in the sink, thus using the full weight of your arm and body for pressure. Many people prefer to work in the sink from the point of view of clearing up any mess afterwards, too.

If you have difficulty in picking up the teapot there are two kinds of stands which help to tip the pot without lifting it. You can even do so without holding its handle. One housewife who finds lifting difficult has had a block made on which to stand her electric kettle, so that she can place the teapot underneath, and tilt the kettle without lifting it. Even for filling the kettle need not be moved, since this can be done either with a jug or

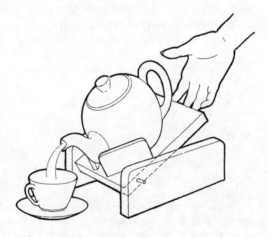

Figure 31.

by using a hose on the tap.

There is not much ordinary cutlery on the market that takes into consideration problems of holding, picking up and weight. The most suitable are the steak sets with wooden handles. Those who need lightweight tools may find plastic picnic cutlery and cups or glasses useful. A cheese knife with a curved blade (the "rocking" principle) and prongs on the end to pick up the food when it is cut is helpful.

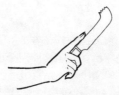

Figure 32.

If your grip is weak larger handles on cutlery are an asset. Pad these with, for example, rubber tubing. If you are unable to lift your arms easily long-handled cutlery, preferably with a gutter for the thumb, is more suitable. Cutlery that is angled so that the spoon or fork reaches your mouth without a twist of the wrist is a help if your wrists are stiff. A cup or mug with a shape in the base to fit your hand makes it difficult to drop and is especially helpful if your hands are unsteady. It is also wise not to fill the cup more than half full.

Clothes and Dressing

Clothing that is easy to manage, comfortable and attractive is a great morale booster. Garments selected by the multiple sclerotic should be styled to:
- reduce stress in dressing and undressing
- counteract the wearing effect of braces, crutches and wheelchair manoeuvering on material
- be comfortable

- be easy to care for
- look attractive

Clothes must have enough "give" to allow the freedom of action necessary to safely propel a wheelchair. Roll-up or short sleeves and flared skirts are more comfortable and less hazardous than long, full designs for wheelchair locomotion. Clothes must be hard-wearing, reinforced at seams, ends of openings and places where extensive abrasion occurs.

Comfort is inherent in the style, size and material. A garment should be cut so that it does not inhibit functioning. This may occasionally necessitate a larger size. Natural fibres are preferable to any other, in particular rough materials and fabrics with static electricity that rub against sensitive skin.

Some of the problems multiple sclerotics encounter can be attenuated by suitable clothing. Smooth-soled shoes which slide over carpets impede a dragging foot the least. A protective covering on the toecaps prevents scuffing. Shoes which give some support but have adjustable fastenings, such as laces or a strap and buckle are essential for legs and feet that swell. When this happens, self-supporting stockings and socks with an elasticised band around the top are to be avoided. Similarly, tight or constricting garments are undesirable if there is any lack of sensation, as are buttons down the back of dresses and hard, bulky seams that may cause pressure.

When sight is severely affected, either choose clothes without fastenings or large, easily grasped buttons, hooks or zips. Buttons and buttonholes in a different colour from the fabric of the garment are more easily seen. Fabrics textured on one side provide another guide to easier dressing for the poorly sighted.

Difficulties with hands — tremor and poor coordination of movements, for example — are lessened where garments are without fastenings: elastic waisted skirts, pullovers, tunics, pinafores and casual open blouses. Marks and stains caused by unavoidable spilling are less noticeable if an all-over patterned fabric is worn. Select knitted cuffs or adapt cuff-buttons with elastic thread.

Light, loose garments with large armholes and openings, or raglan sleeves facilitate dressing and undressing where there is general weakness of the upper limbs. Beach shirts, overblouses and long tunics prevent unsightly gaps at the waist and allow unrestricted shoulder movement to crutch-users. Waist seams tend to ride up and become torn, but loose A-line or pinafore dresses are comfortable and stay in place. Pockets are very necessary but neither they nor any other trimming should protrude to obstruct your view of the ground.

Plenty of room across the back of the shoulders is essential for self-propelled wheelchair-users. Long, full sleeves and skirts tend to catch in the wheel spokes and short coats should reach only to the seat of the chair.

If independence cannot be achieved by the careful selection of style and fastening alone, it may be necessary to adopt a new method of dressing with or without the use of certain aids.

Many are designed to alleviate the problems arising from restricted reach, and their selection depends on the extent of the limitation. Several devices can extend reach and grasp but require some movement and power of the fingers. A simple dressing stick is also useful to hook clothes over feet and shoulders. This can be improvised from a coat hanger: remove the centre hook and add a rubber thimble to one end and a small, brass screw hook to the other.

When learning to dress try not to become overtired or frustrated; tackle the easiest garments and fastenings first. Undressing is simpler than dressing, so begin with taking off a blouse, then proceed to lower extremity clothes and finally to fastenings.

Upper extremity dressing need not be unduly difficult for multiple sclerotics. At the start, place all garments within reach, arranged in order of dressing. Any horizontal surface which supports the elbows, either when sitting or standing, can help you pull clothes over your head if your shoulders are stiff. When one arm (or leg) is weaker or stiffer than the other, put the affected limb in the garment first and remove it last. For example, first insert your weaker arm into the sleeve of a blouse and push it on up the shoulder; then either throw the garment over your shoulder and round the back, or hook it around with a dressing stick; insert your other arm and fasten.

Weakness, ataxia and easy fatigue often make lower extremity dressing very awkward. Dressing on a bed gives support for your whole body, keeps the clothes from falling, engenders a feeling of stability and enables you to reach your feet without bending down. Light suspender belts and pull-ons can be pulled over head or feet. Roll from side to side on the bed to ease the garment into position. Any long-reaching device can hook a skirt over the feet; it is then pulled up by rolling the body from one side to the other.

To put on socks or stockings, sit on the side of the bed that must be low enough to allow both feet to be placed firmly on the ground. If you have a tendency to fall to one side, place a chair alongside the bed to support the weaker side. Now either lift your foot onto a low stool or cross one knee over the other. If you have difficulty bending, use a high release device made from a stick, tape and a suspender end. Loops sewn on the tops of socks may also be helpful.

Slip-on shoes without fastenings are the most appropriate if feet do not swell and if ankles are stiff, as often happens in multiple sclerosis. Where there is difficulty in reaching the feet, the soft back of a slipper tends to double over when it is put on. To overcome this, stitch a small loop to the back of the slipper and hook it with a dressing stick.

Communication Aids

Electronic technology has made significant strides in recent years, simplifying life for the handicapped and home-bound. In multiple sclerosis with a wide variation in the degree of disability, the versatility of electronic technology is stretched to the limit. In the majority of cases even the most severely disabled person with the disease can be helped to lead a more independent life.

Severe physical disability does not mean mental inability and generally the brain remains an intelligent, thinking, controlling force, but with nothing to control. This realisation led to the development in England of a range of systems for controlling electronically what the body was unable to physically.

These systems are called "Possum" which means, in Latin, "I can" and originates from the letters P.O.S.M. (Patient Operated Selector Mechanisms).

Possum™ equipment is a wide range of electronic aids enabling severely physically disabled people to exercise efficient and effortless control over domestic, commercial and industrial equipment. The systems are operated by mouth (pneumatic switch — independent of respiratory breathing) or, where there is some residual physical ability — just a flicker in a finger — by a microswitch or a set of these.

The systems are broadly divided into three categories: environmental controls, keyboard-operated apparatus, and all types of communication equipment. The one most widely used is the Possum Selector Unit Type 1. This gives independence in the home and control over the immediate environment. It allows a disabled person to select and switch on/off up to eleven electrical devices, such as an emergency and nonemergency calling system (bell and buzzer), heat, light, radio, TV and intercom system to door and electric door lock, and a loudspeaking telephone. The telephone control gives full self-dialing facility and control over the volume.

Technical aids not only help the handicapped person by extending independence, however. More important perhaps, is the peace of mind and reduction in stress they afford to family and friends. But for every person who needs such sophisticated environmental control, there are many times that number whose disability is less severe and are able to benefit from simpler and less costly items of equipment. There are those who simply require a console of switches to operate alarm, intercom link with the front door and perhaps one or two other electrical functions. There is also a self-contained intercom link with the front door which is battery operated. This unit is light to carry and many multiple sclerotics find units like these of tremendous value, eliminating the need to leave keys in the door or hanging on a string through the letterbox.

By plugging the units of a special wireless intercom into the appropriate mains power outlet, communication by voice and alarm signal from room to room and, where necessary, from house to house is possible. On occasion communication from house to house over a distance of several hundred yards has been achieved.

Moving away from electronic technology, the telephone has proven to be the most effective and easiest communication aid for the multiple sclerotic to manage. The use of the standard telephone requires coordination among many muscles and joints in the upper extremity. Deficits in auditory sensation, speech, perception and sight, as well as incoordination and decreased muscle strength, can complicate normal use of the telephone. Amplifying handsets help to offset auditory defects, much as poor sight is assisted by large-print books or a magnifying glass.

The position of the phone for the most comfortable and efficient use is the first consideration. This is especially important when reach is limited and space at a premium. Extension cords of varied lengths and extension brackets which extend the phone from its resting surface are valuable in this regard. There are numerous other aids which overcome the inability to hold the handset. Pain, weakness or loss of fine finger movements as well as generalised upper extremity involvement may make dialing difficult if not impossible to perform. Dialing aids range from the substitution of a pencil for finger to the automatic dialers now on the market.

Individuals with limited upper extremity function are sometimes partially or completely unable to cope with the dynamics involved in reading. Strength and grasp may be insufficient to support the weight of a book, coordination may be so impaired that the individual is unable to turn pages. More work has been done on the development of page turning equipment than almost any other facet of aids for the handicapped. Many designs have been produced but so far most have drawbacks. The wide variety of different books (hardback, paperback, various sizes and textures of paper, etc.) make the possibility of a really versatile page turner somewhat remote. However, an electrically operated page turner is now available which can be triggered by a single microswitch, or even by a light puff down a tube, and it will turn both hard- and paperbacks.

Any activity that requires maintaining muscles in one position for long periods of time tends to increase fatigue. Thus the book should never be held, but rested instead in a propped position. With a reading stand, the muscles of the upper extremity relax, reducing muscle fatigue and joint discomfort. Inexpensive book holders of wire or wood may be made at home or purchased.

Mass media devices such as radio and television are among the major contacts with the world around us, and are especially important to the multiple sclerotic. Slight hand involvement may affect one's ability to turn knobs, limited range of movement may necessitate special placement of the appliance, and severe involvement may require remote control or specially designed apparatus. In selecting a model, look for raised front controls as they are easiest to manage when there is weakness or incoordination in the upper extremity. Large, easily rotated knobs with ridged outer surfaces provide more friction for turning.

Employment

There is little doubt that employers are unwilling to engage people disabled or handicapped through multiple sclerosis. Unfortunately, the reasons for their reluctance are valid. Multiple sclerosis is an unpredictable disease. A sufferer can have one episode or a dozen in a lifetime, each affecting different parts of the body. She can have remissions which are partial or complete, the illness can be progressive or remain stable; in short, the future is unpredictable.

In practical terms uncertainty means unreliability, a particularly unattractive trait to a prospective employer. How can he know when, how often and for how long the multiple sclerotic might have to request sick leave, and what guarantee is there that she will be able to fulfill the same job afterwards?

Equally unfortunate, in our society appraisal of the individual's achievement is ultimately vocational. Thus the multiple sclerotic whose disease frequently begins in the teens and early twenties, may not ever have the opportunity to be measured by this yardstick. Of course, many sufferers are able to continue their careers unscathed, but others are plagued by both practical and attitudinal problems. Every advantage must be taken of the person's educational and vocational background to redirect her skills into an avenue compatible with her physical abilities.

The development of a career is probably dictated as much by the flexibility of the one chosen as by the disease and the attitude of employers. Medicine, for example, has a large degree of flexibility: doctors, who are especially prone to multiple sclerosis, can move from extremely demanding positions to those involving lighter duties; nurses can go from wards and theatres to community clinics, reception work and so on.

Multiple sclerosis can reduce stamina, mobility or both. When mobility is impaired, accessibility becomes of paramount importance. In either case, however, further education or retraining may be necessary and possible for the sufferer. Electronic systems, such as Possum, also provide a means for the professional or businesswoman to return either to previous or new employment.

Undoubtedly, a satisfactory and rewarding working life with multiple sclerosis is possible. Sufferers are often advised to aim high and to convince employers, if necessary, of their suitability to the job in question. If changes are necessary they adapt as required, never lose their optimistic approach, and apparently find that employers tend to take their cue from them.

This approach and attitude may be admirable for the majority. However, it could be that work and career have an etiologic link, direct or indirect, with multiple sclerosis. The relation between a person and any situation is a dialogue. Sometimes in industrial society the dialogue becomes a disputation which, in conjunction with other factors, leads to breakdown and disease. Perhaps multiple sclerosis is the opportunity some of us need to reexamine our lives, in particular our work; to grieve its loss where this is inevitable; and then to seek, to find and to develop a new direction wherein the forces of our lives can be more wholesomely integrated. Many of us would not voluntarily relinquish the rat race of the modern world;

maybe we should be grateful not heartbroken, when some untoward event forces us to reconsider the course we have chosen, or been pushed into, and then perhaps we should ensure that the benefits we gain from any fresh insights are permanent.

Leisure-time activities

Leisure time can be spent productively to maintain and develop increased intellectual and other functioning, and self-esteem. There are many activities available for the moderately to severely handicapped which are often therapeutic as well as interesting and challenging:

Gardening and indoor horticulture
Reading or talking books
Handicrafts
Listening to music
Creative writing

Such activities have the potential to deflect the sufferer from concentrating upon her disability and toward a worthy productiveness that can enhance life, her's and those of people around her.

Physical Therapy

Physical therapy is aimed at improving or preventing the consequences and varied complications of multiple sclerosis. The time for it is when the disease appears to be relatively stable or retrogressing. It builds up muscular strength and functional capacity which, in turn, increase the individual's ability to perform her activities of daily living.

No single regimen is suitable for all sufferers. No two are alike, so no two treatments are the same. Every program is appropriately tailored to the individual's medical status, needs and problems. Very few generalisations are applicable but an almost universal maxim is to avoid muscle fatigue. In multiple sclerosis fatigue lessens motor power for a longer period of time and to a greater degree than is usually seen in other illnesses.

The use of heat is also avoided as it may cause a severe exacerbation and even bring to light unsuspected subclinical deficits. These are usually reversible.

Decreased motor power is a significantly disabling feature of multiple sclerosis. The distribution of weakness follows no set pattern. It may affect a single extremity, both lower extremities, three or all four extremities, or both extremities on the same side. The sufferer may describe her symptoms only as easy fatigability or a feeling of heaviness. The loss of motor power actually caused by the disease is *not* reversed by exercises or any other physical modality. What real weakness there is, however, may be accompanied by the weakness of disuse resulting from long periods of immobilisation. For this reason strengthening exercises may be tried judiciously, always avoiding damaging fatigue.

Another disabling feature is spasticity with or without weakness. Spasticity alone, even in its mildest form, can be a deterrent to function, particularly gait. It is often possible to learn certain techniques to overcome or circumvent this defect.

In the more severe stage of spasticity, irreversible shortening of muscles with consequent contracture of joints may occur. Now the maintenance of joint mobility can no longer be accomplished by activity on the part of the multiple sclerotic, but must be effected through passive exercises. A family member, friend or the home nurse can learn to carry these out daily to minimise joint contractures.

One other manifestation of weakness and spasticity often seen in multiple sclerosis is ataxia and incoordination. One of the functions of the cerebellum of the brain is to smooth and integrate impulses from the cerebrum. With cerebellar activity diminished, as it may be in multiple sclerosis, this integrated motion breaks down into its component parts resulting in observable jerkiness and clumsiness of motion (ataxia). It may be seen in one or all extremities or in the trunk. Gait training can be beneficial. Sometimes just widening the base of support increases stability sufficiently to permit safe ambulation. In other cases, a crutch, cane or walker may be needed for that purpose.

Incoordination in the upper extremities may be of such a degree as to preclude the use of these aids. There are several simple self-help devices which are useful in overcoming this incoordination in uncomplicated activities of daily living. Weighted bracelets or cuffs on the wrists or ankles may help by diminishing excursion of the ataxia. Weighted eating utensils facilitate self-feeding in these cases. However, the overall success in the management of ataxia leaves much to be desired.

Among the cranial nerves affected by multiple sclerosis, perhaps the most frequently involved are the optic nerves, the several ocular motor nerves and the nerves controlling mechanisms of speech. Treatment has not been successful in altering the various scotoma and/or blindness sometimes seen in multiple sclerosis. In many instances of diplopia (double vision), there is suppression of one of the images after several months of illness, so that this is not a long-term problem. The most effective way of dealing with diplopia, even at the cost of some depth perception, is to obscure visual impulses into one eye by a patch or frosted lens. It is far better to see a single image lacking depth than to face the confusion of double images.

Dysarthia (impairment of articulation) marked by low volume of speech, slurring, incoordinative phonation, and scanning of syllables, is common. Progressive resistive exercises can be given to the muscles of phonation such as the muscles of respiration, tongue and face. Rhythm and rapidity of speech have been less responsive to treatment than volume and pronunciation.

Many patterns of sensory loss are recognised in multiple sclerosis. Precautions must be taken to avoid trauma to the skin from heat, cold, pressure and other noxious agents. There has been little success in restoring sensation. The Pifco™ vibrator, which imparts a vibratory motor stimulus, can be used safely throughout the day and seems to help those with slight sensory defects, especially in hands and feet. The use of a stimulator should never serve to make the muscle tone abnormal, i.e. render someone who is hypertonic more spastic, and should be followed by exercises to improve coordination once sensory awareness is greater.

Hand-eye coordinated movements can be trained so that even with an insensitive hand you can learn from visual appreciation the correct degrees of pressure to be exerted on objects to be manipulated.

Professor Russell has developed, and claimed success for, a program of rest and exercise (REP). It is based on the theory that the lesions in multiple sclerosis are caused, or influenced by, areas of circulatory insufficiency in the white matter of the central nervous system, and that these areas would be less likely to appear if the circulatory system were maintained in the robust state of the trained athlete.

The exercises to improve coordination of spasms of limbs which make up a program of physical therapy are a separate issue. Russell believes that they are less important than the REP. This, too, must be adapted to the type of disability; if the multiple sclerotic is not disabled, running, skipping, cycling, sports, gardening or exercise on a rowing machine is added to the daily plan.

Russell advises short periods (10-20 minutes) of rest, lying down two to three times during the day. Before, during or after this period any type of "mat exercise" is undertaken. The most vigorous part of the exercises is done with the upper limbs. This encourages a response in the blood circulation of the upper spinal cord and brain stem. There are many suitable types of arm exercises for this purpose, for example, press-ups, weight lifting and use of springs. The effort is intended to cause flushing of the face, head and neck, and acceleration of heart rate. This program is to be carried out daily for the rest of the multiple sclerotic's life.

The Facts of Being Multiple Sclerotic

In Sickness and in Health . . .

Marriage for the handicapped falls into three different categories. There is marriage between two disabled people; marriage between an able-bodied person and someone disabled; and marriage between two able-bodied people, one of whom becomes disabled later through a sudden accident or disease. When a disabled couple — or a couple, one of whom is disabled — decide to marry or live their lives together, a good deal of thinking has to be done in advance. It may be necessary to decide who carries out the household chores, who is to be the main breadwinner, or how these roles can be shared. Possible sexual difficulties need to be explored. The couple may have to adopt a quite different life-style from that of able-bodied people, and to feel comfortable in it.

When disability through multiple sclerosis occurs after marriage, a similar situation may have to be faced. First, there is the tremendous anxiety over the disease and its unpredictable course. Perhaps the only way to cope with this is by working through the grief consequent upon the diagnosis and then living and enjoying life day by day, dealing with each problem as it arises and not fretting about those that may never materialise. Secondly, whichever partner is affected, there is likely to be financial strain through loss of income or pin-money, and medical expenses. Thirdly, the social life of a multiple sclerotic couple has to be curtailed. Clearly, impaired mobility and easy fatigability make outings anywhere more difficult and can lead to physical isolation. However, your disability cannot always be blamed for this. If you do not regard your altered appearance as too important and if you do not withdraw from other people, the chances are that others will not be off-hand with you. Retaining old friends and making new ones means effort on your part but is certainly not impossible.

The outlook of both partners on disability itself is important. Some people are not worried by handicap or bodily difference, others find certain kinds of disability repellant. The multiple lesions in multiple sclerosis may be distributed throughout the white matter of the cerebrum, the cerebellum and brain stem, as well as the spinal cord. Inevitably there is often a wide variety of emotional reactions. Euphoria is a characteristic change in the affect of many sufferers, but so are devastating depressions, disorganised anxiety states, self-destructive acts, antisocial behavior, aggressive and dependency states, all important psychologic barriers to *any* effective interpersonal relationship. In short, you may seem to be another person due to the invisible lesions in your nervous system. Your husband may feel that you have changed beyond recognition and find it hard to be both nurse and lover. The real self within you is suppressed and forced to give way to the all-consuming disability which the world sees and so readily rejects.

As one spastic put it: "For as long as I can remember I have been conscious of two me's — the outer casing which is visible to the world and the inner substance which is not. The outer casing is of course my body and is the facade which, in all but a few circumstances, the world judges me. The inner part is my mind, my character, my conscience and my true being. Take away my twisted limbs, peel off my peculiar facial expressions and remove all traces of my athetoid condition and you will be left with a normal man."[37]

With the onset of severe or prolonged symptoms, demanding more of your husband's time and effort, your marriage may be subjected to a strong tendency toward disintegration. He may feel anger at your dependence and then guilt about feeling angry. If his interests shift elsewhere, psychologic isolation compounds the frustration and guilt you feel because of your sense of inadequacy and inequality in the marriage. To some extent the unwelcome burdens you are forced to inflict on your husband can be offset by revitalising and giving full expression to those essential aspects of a close marital bond: support, warmth, patience, love and a genuine sense of caring.

Unless you are euphoric, achieving the acceptance that allows you to be of good cheer most of the time, is a tough and never-ending battle. But the fight could pay dividends since many men can take in their stride the additional responsibilities of a wife incurably ill with a capricious disease; what they cannot tolerate, and eventually seek to escape, is that despite their best efforts their partners always seem to be miserable.

A central aspect of every woman's personality is her sexuality. This is more than simply a physiologic experience; it includes the psychologic, social and interpersonal aspects of every woman. It is logical to assume therefore, that even a serious physical disability does not eliminate sexual needs, although it is likely to interrupt a normal sexual relationship between you and your husband.

It is natural to experience all sorts of doubts, anxieties and fears regarding sexuality. The physical symptoms of the disease affect your body image and view of yourself as sexually attractive and desirable; they shatter all feelings of femaleness. They also may make intercourse difficult. Conflict between your sexual desires and your ability, physically and psychologically, to fulfill them is probably unavoidable.

If sexual adjustment is difficult for a relatively healthy woman, it is obviously more difficult for one with a serious debilitative disease, and for her husband. If communication about sexual feelings is difficult within a relationship in which both partners are physically healthy, it will be more difficult when the woman has physical problems which interfere with sexual expression and gratification.

A woman who is multiple sclerotic may be frigid due perhaps to numbness or other sensory disturbance in the clitoris and vagina. In this case, stimulation of the clitoris and vagina either prior to or during intercourse will produce neither secretions nor orgasm. This may mean unsatisfactory sexual relations for both partners; however, as sensory symptoms are often temporary, so is frigidity.

One problem a woman may experience is intense adductor spasm in the thighs (muscular fixing and cramping which brings the legs together, sometimes very tightly). Severely spastic adductor muscles create a mechanical barrier to intercourse, as well as in positioning for delivery. Adductor spasm also interferes with personal hygiene and walking. A variety of neurosurgical and orthopedic procedures are available for the relief of this state.

Most women with multiple sclerosis continue to menstruate. This usually means that they are continuing to ovulate; and where the disease can be controlled, pregnancy is neither impossible nor always inadvisable. It does sometimes cause some decompensation of bowel control and bladder function. But this may also occur in normal women who, of course, are better equipped to deal with problems of frequency or urgency. Labour in itself is no problem whatsoever.

The main anxiety about pregnancy is its likely effect on the course of the disease. Doctors are either reluctant to commit themselves on this issue or else tend to firmly oppose the proposal to have a baby. The reason is the generally accepted fact that while pregnancy itself may not affect the disease, there is some increase in relapses during the postnatal months, their magnitude depending on the mother's condition. This increase is attributed to the stress of labour as well as the additional work and responsibility involved. Less generally known, is that allergic manifestations are accentuated following pregnancy.

Any decision about family planning naturally leads to the choice of a contraceptive. Even today disabled couples are diffident about asking for contraceptive advice; at the back of their minds there is always the feeling that they should not be having sex at all. Whichever method is chosen, the main point is that it should be as safe as possible, because few couples can afford mistakes. If it does fail, termination of pregnancy probably would not be refused to a handicapped woman. Nevertheless an abortion is an experience most women would prefer to avoid. The disabled woman who has chosen to remain childless may find it very difficult to agree to an abortion once she finds she is pregnant. She may have made a rational decision not to have children, but she will feel very torn if she has to make a decision because of a mistake. So although abortion can bring relief, it also brings grief to many.

In the face of religious or other beliefs which prohibit contraception it may help to see its practise not so much as a way of stopping children, but as a means of achieving a happy life together without increasing the burden of your handicap. You can then enjoy sex for what it is, and your relationship with each other, without the fear of bringing children into the world.

If your husband has multiple sclerosis his potential for intercourse depends on the nature of the lesions in the nervous system. Men with partial upper motor neuron lesions may be capable of sexual functions and about 10 percent of siring children. In these cases there is perineal sensation; that is, in the penis, scrotum and hind saddle area; muscle tone, particularly of the anal sphincter, is preserved; and the pelvic muscles can be voluntarily contracted.

Men so affected may differ from normal in that an erection depends on mechanical or tactile stimulation of the skin of the pelvis, lower abdomen, or some other part of the body, and the erections may be fleeting. If they do not last very long or are inhibited, intercourse is obviously disrupted. A few men with partial upper motor neuron lesions fail to achieve erection. Nevertheless, they are able, mechanically at least, to initiate intercourse; some are capable of completing it, even though the act may require considerable postural adjustment of the partners. A small proportion have erections in response to psychologic events or during sleep. In addition, ejaculation is often absent or delayed; if, as a result, intercourse is very prolonged, injury to the urethra may occur. Some time limit on intercourse should therefore be set.

Generally speaking, if there is sensation, good muscle tone and some degree of voluntary movement, and the man still cannot have intercourse, it is highly probable that his impotence has a strong psychogenic component. If you suspect that this is so, do not make the disease your scapegoat; examine your attitudes towards sex as well as the marital relationship as a whole. Jealousy, resentment, anger, insecurity and feelings of inferiority can prevent and block the communication that should take place during intercourse. Sex is a means of telling your partner your feelings, your love and your joys; of sharing a deep pool of real individuality. It is despicable to use the disease as a decoy for pathology within the marriage which, under normal circumstances, would lead to divorce.

No sexual practice, provided it is enjoyed by both partners and harms no one, can reasonably be regarded as abnormal or bad.[62,90] If loving and sex are to be at their best, both partners must help each other. Some people are shy about trying out new ideas or practices, or even discussing them with their partners. But talking matters over together and experimenting with possible solutions can be very worthwhile. There is one golden rule: love and patience on the part of both seldom fails to solve problems. Husband and wife should tell each other what they like (or do not like). They should encourage each other, never criticise. But each must be able to make the other confident enough to seek, with reasonable consideration, his or her own pleasure, knowing that this is the best way to help both.

The variety of positions and techniques for sex is rarely exploited. Because they may differ from those you are accustomed to, this does not mean that there is anything wrong with them or that you are kinky if you try them. Any position which gives pleasure to both and which hurts neither is good. It is seldom that at least one position which is comfortable and pleasant cannot be found. There are excellent books of photographs which most couples will find useful. There is always value in reading sex books together, for they encourage communication by offering a framework of mutual experience, even if it is only visual. In exploring new positions, it may be necessary to try several and to spend a little time in practice. This may well prove to be a rewarding investment.

If a sexual difficulty is not solved by adopting a different position, perhaps a better knowledge of the diverse methods of sexual intercourse will be of help. Provided these are undertaken with love and warmth, and are not seen as a distasteful chore, sex can still be enjoyable and satisfying.

Numerous improvised or artificial aids can be used to resolve sexual difficulties. These vary from such everyday articles as pillows or cushions to specially made appliances. Adduction, for example, may be overcome by placing a firm cushion below the woman's hips and another between her legs to support her body in a suitable position. Heavy cushions or pads can often reduce muscular spasms in the legs.

The manufactured aids are often regarded with suspicion and those who use them as dirty and sinful; experimentation is a retrograde step along the steep slope to licentiousness and hell. Yet we do not hesitate to wear glasses if we want to see better and few people would refuse, if it became necessary, to accept an artificial limb. Why jib at aids designed to improve sex?

A Roman Catholic priest wrote to a magazine recently about a parishioner of his, a young man of eighteen, who had been involved in a serious road accident and was now paralysed from the waist down. He was impotent. During his convalescence he became friendly with a healthy girl of his own age. They fell in love. The priest felt that marriage between them could nevertheless still be wonderfully satisfying.

"They are so involved with each other and so much in love," he wrote, "that a break would be shattering for them both, but especially for the boy who has already suffered so much. I feel that provided he accepts with some grace the fact that there can be no more sexual satisfaction for him and provided she accepts that she will not be able to have his children, I believe their future together could be good. Sexual fulfillment for her will be limited and for him the satisfactions of the marriage will be on another level. I believe normal sexual intercourse could be simulated by the boy wearing an artificial penis, and masturbation and oral sex can all play a part in their relationship."[37]

The priest was right on target. Artificial aids provide an extra dimension to the sex lives of many people, disabled or able-bodied. They can help handicapped people to achieve a level of emotional independence and satisfaction to which they have every right, but which every societal agency, from parents downwards, seem bent on denying them. So long as we imply that there is some shame involved, the handicapped will either be refused access to these aids, including books labelled by the watchdogs of public morals as pornographic, or have their enjoyment, if and when they do get them, ruined by feelings of guilt.

Even where intercourse is really out of the question, lovemaking in other ways is pleasant — by using the hands, for instance. Touching is good and pleasurable, and if it is done in a loving and sensitive manner, the relief provided can be considerable and the experience a joy. Where no feeling exists in the sexual organs, other parts of the body often increase in sexual feeling. Stroking and caressing of the breasts, neck and other parts of the body can give delight. When feeling is lost below a certain level of the body that part immediately above it sometimes becomes hypersensitive.

The key to adjustment between any multiple sclerotic couple

is communication. The partners must make as many opportunities as they need to discuss with each other their feelings. Talking about things, laughing about them, however wryly, helps to relieve tension and keep problems well in perspective. Putting those very personal feelings into words and deeds helps a couple to understand and appreciate each other, to grow as individuals, and the marriage to develop into something deep and lasting. Conversely, if they are not dealt with, frustrated feelings can lead to hostility and ultimately, a complete breakdown of the relationship. The saddest event in the life of any multiple sclerotic is the loss of a spouse through the inept handling of the strains and stresses caused by the state of being multiple sclerotic.

... *To Be or Not to Be?*

> Everyman is endowed at birth by his parents and ancestors with a type of constitution built of anatomical, physiological, immunological and psychological material which will help to determine his course through life and his reactions to environmental stress and injury.
>
> —J. A. Ryle

Various areas of concern relate to the decision to have a child or not. First, there is the possibility of handing down the disability to him. There is frequent confusion between terms when we talk about genetic disease. *Congenital* applied to a particular disease or abnormality means only that it is present at birth. It has no causal or etiologic connotation. Congenital abnormalities may be due to environmental factors, e.g. thalidomide or rubella infection, to pure genetic factors, e.g. gene or chromosomal defects, or to the interaction between these. A *familial* disease runs in families and, again, may be the product of genes, chromosomes and/or environmental factors. It is a descriptive rather than an etiologic term. *Hereditary* refers to traits transmitted by direct descent from an affected member of a family to his/her offspring. The term is a synonym for *genetic*.

Human characteristics are always the result of an interaction between genetic factors and environmental influences. Most disease has some genetic component, of variable importance, in its etiology. Human diseases range on a spectrum from those that are predominently environmental in origin, e.g. lead poisoning or infections, to others that are entirely genetic (mongolism or haemophilia). Between these extremes are many common diseases such as hypertension and diabetes mellitus, and congenital abnormalities like spina bifida where the genetic component is modified by different environmental factors.

Genetic disease is classified into three general groups: those associated with abnormalities of the chromosomes; those due to a single abnormal gene or abnormal gene pair; and those resulting from the interaction of several abnormal genes, each with small detrimental effects, and environmental influences, known as multifactorial conditions.

In recent years a familial tendency to multiple sclerosis has been generally recognised: that is, a minority of families have a constitutional vulnerability to the disease. Familial studies carried out in a number of countries suggest that the proportion of first degree living relatives of multiple sclerotics is about fifteen to twenty times that expected. The incidence of multiple sclerosis in relatives in descending order of frequency is: siblings, parents, children, other relatives.

Conditions that run in families have polygenic characteristics. This means they are due to a complex interaction of both hereditary and environmental factors, and the extent of the hereditary component varies from one condition to the other; they are multifactorial in that they involve a number of different hereditary and environmental influences; the hereditary component is polygenic; it consists of a number of minor genes, each making a small contribution to produce a large effect; clinical manifestations depend on a strong genetic predisposition that puts the individual at a point of risk where environmental influences determine whether (and in some cases to what extent) he/she will be affected. In short, two factors determine whether or not the signs and symptoms of multiple sclerosis appear: (1) a familial or genetic tendency to the disease; (2) environmental stress.

If you are concerned about handing down your disease, discuss the matter with your general practitioner. Better still, seek specialist advice in the form of genetic counselling. This deals with the human problems associated with the occurrence, or risk of occurrence, of a genetic disorder in a family. The counsellor tries to help the family comprehend the medical facts, including the diagnosis, the probable course of the disorder, and the available management; to appreciate the way heredity contributes to the disorder, and the risk of recurrence in specified relatives; to understand the options for dealing with the risk of recurrence; to choose the course of action that seems appropriate to them in light of their risk and family goals and to act accordingly; and, finally, to make the best possible adjustment to the disorder in an affected family member and/or to the risk of its recurrence.

The mode of inheritance determines the degree of risk related to the disease. As a general rule, the more definite and clear-cut the genetics, the greater the risks; as the genetics become more obscure, the outlook becomes more hopeful. The recurrence risks for heritable disorders also fall into three groups. First, those in which there is more or less the same random risk for *any* pregnancy in the population; this is in the order of one in thirty. Secondly, those where there is a high risk of one in ten or greater and last, those with a moderate risk of fewer than one in ten. The largest proportion of genetic disorders is in this category. Included are all those conditions that "run in families." But although a genetic element is present in these disorders, there is no clear-cut affected-unaffected classification.

When the laws of inheritance are applied to polygenic characteristics, the expectation is that relatives will have more genes in common. Thus there is an increased likelihood that these will be expressed more often when united with a similar combination of genes. If the gene/s is common, relatives will receive it from different sources; if it is rare, they will seldom inherit it. The more distant the relationship, the fewer genes that are shared.

The risk of recurrence in multifactorial-polygenic inheritance is less than one in ten but substantially greater than the random risk in the population as a whole. Risk estimates by the genetic counsellor of your child developing multiple sclerosis are *empiric;* that is, estimates are based not on genetic theory but on prior experience and observation, much the same as the grounds on which a meterologist makes a weather prediction. To determine an empiric risk, the counsellor applies a knowledge of the frequencies observed in families with a similar condition to the incidence of the disorder in your family. Since his prediction is only an estimate based on incidence in other families, his figures are likely to be exaggerated in some families and underestimated in others.

In giving you a risk estimate the genetic counsellor is neither making nor implying recommendations or decisions. All he is able to give you is reliable information about the nature of the disorder, the probable extent of the risk involved and the consequences insofar as he can assess them. The final decision to have a child or not is entirely your own affair.

From a psychologic point of view, the handicapped mother must make an enormous effort to cope adequately. Her success depends largely on, first, a realistic appraisal of the many dimensions of the undertaking. To begin with, the home circumstances of a mother who is multiple sclerotic are probably less than ideal. Understandably, the multiple sclerotic is often more sensitive about this than others who, in fact, have equal cause for concern, but never give the matter a thought. How many homes do you know that are ideal? Working mothers are accused of neglecting their primary duty; travelling fathers are said to inflict stresses upon their offspring; in many marriages children are forced to witness quarrel after quarrel; the hectic social life of so many couples is hardly compatible with their children's welfare. The list could be extended indefinitely.

At the least the handicapped mother is aware that her circumstances are not perfect. In consequence, however, she must be willing, and able, to elicit help from others. This is really only one more area where the interdependence of *all* human beings is amplified by being multiple sclerotic. The complex transformation of a biologic creature into a psychologic being emphasizes the importance of our sociocultural environment, although the volumes of popular psychology on child care scarcely give this impression. Instead mothers are bludgeoned with the necessity for unremitting love on their part and the dire effects of even short separations from their infant, all neatly rationalised by the threat to the infant of "maternal deprivation." The essence of maternal deprivation — it has even been accorded the status of theory — is that the unbroken care of one mother is vital to every infant, not just for its immediate well-being and contentment, but for his future mental and emotional health.

To a remarkable extent, this belief has shaped social attitudes in western countries since World War II, elevating motherhood to a position of awesome responsibility compounded of skill, dedication and psychologic insight. Today's mother doubts the ability of her child's school, peer-group, friends or relatives to help her provide any of the elementary lessons about the world and life. Instead she has been convinced that she, and she alone, is responsible for whether he grows up intelligent or dull, emotionally developed or immature and repressed, loving and cooperative or affectionless and hating everyone in sight. It is difficult to think of any kind of infant, child, adolescent or adult deviance for which mothers have escaped censure.

Actually there is no reason at all why we ought to believe that maternal deprivation — a phrase, incidentally, that defies definition — really does have irreversibly detrimental effects on later personality development. The firm conviction that it does stems from psychoanalysis which is speculative to say the least, having no more empirical support than palmistry or astrology. One of the most invidious unproven principles in the psycho-analytic tradition is that any stress in childhood is alien and potentially traumatising and that any momentary unhappiness can be construed as stress.

The mooted etiologic connection between maternal depriva-tion and personality damage has no significant scientific basis and sufficient counter-evidence to make it decidedly improbable. It would be a great mistake therefore for the woman who is multiple sclerotic to be persuaded against having a child *on the basis of* a radically misleading view of child psychology. This peculiar a-cultural view of childhood has caused misery enough, for example by forcing children to remain in control of violent, cruel or hopelessly negligent parents, without also adding unnecessarily to the chronic uncertainties of being multiple sclerotic. Rather it is considerations like the extent of the disability, the husband's earning capacity, as well as the personality of both parents that must carry the most weight in coming to a decision about having a child.

The basic assumption behind the idea of maternal deprivation is that important individual qualities are formed in the child during sensitive periods in his first five years of life. The nurturing of this embryo personality is so entwined with the mother's biologic presence and processes that it cannot be delegated. But genetic predispositions aside, these qualities of competence, compassion, responsibility, and moral understanding cannot be created by any process of individual nurture determined by the child's needs. These qualities depend upon lifelong practice and participation in public communal life as the folkways of any preindustrial society will confirm.

There is an urgent need for widening the guardianship and upbringing of children both in general and with respect to those who, like multiple sclerotics, have special problems to contend with. Some attempt must be made to open up the nuclear family, to share parental functions with people who become involved in one way or another at a fundamental level with children not biologically theirs.

Handicapped mothers are likely to feel especially anxious about separations from their young children through periodic hospitalisation. However, the major cause of distress to the child in these circumstances is probably the amount of change in the total environment, rather than just the absence of his mother. There is little indication in research that upset occurs if a separated child is left at home with his father or grandparents. Similarly, whether the child is left at home or sent away, the presence of siblings also mitigates distress. If the child can stay in the environment he is used to, even though a part of it (in the shape of his mother) goes away, or if he can take some

Multiple Sclerosis

of his social environment with him, e.g. a sibling, anguish is virtually absent.

Accustom your child from an early age to benign separation, so that life is less of a shock later. Encourage him to move outside your immediate family so he can develop social skills useful in a world wider than his home, intelligible to more than one or two adults. While it may not be ideal, why not make use of extrafamilial experiences, such as hospitalisation, as appropriately managed circumstances for your child to acquire some of the learning missed through his sheltered and probably matriarchal early home experience? After the intial upset, a separation can be a valuable experience, leading to maturation and social responsiveness.

Nevertheless, knowing that the first five years need not be permanently crippling does not automatically lighten the burden of child care. But as it is not a biologic process inexplicably connected in some instinctual way with being female, men as well as women can, and should, share in it. And as child care becomes more explicit, so its scope becomes more finite. There is a definite limit to what you or anyone can or cannot do for your child, to the things that can and cannot be achieved. The contemporary wisdom that continually goads every mother, handicapped or not, to worry that her child is not getting enough of vaguely defined attentions; that things may be going wrong inside without any way of really telling; that there is always something more she can do, is a monstrous perversion.

The handicapped mother must also recognise her feelings about her condition and how these affect her relationship with her baby. It helps a great deal to talk about them to friends. She may well experience considerable guilt which can interfere, often severely, in the actual formation of a relationship. A mother may believe herself incapable of caring for and protecting her baby. Even when in contact with him then, she does not dare do much without permission. Guidance in how to hold, dress and feed her infant may be essential to help her overcome her "mothering paralysis." Special reassurance gives her the confidence to get on with her own style of mothering. Her greatest fears occur when her infant comes home; she may even be afraid to feed the baby by herself, or bathe him.

Guilt feelings have a way of smothering any willingness to ask questions. Caring for and socialising a child involves mastery of quite detailed child-care procedures, even for elementary tasks. Like every other skill, child care is culturally acquired. It varies from society to society and it does not come naturally; it is not an instinct which matures in an appropriate emotional atmosphere during the mother's own babyhood some two decades previously. Demanding good child care from untaught, isolated parents is unheard of in any other society.

There is absolutely no reason why handicapped women cannot be taught this skill; multiple sclerosis affects the body and only rarely the mind. Expecting women who are multiple sclerotic to forego the pleasure of children because the limitations of the disease shapes their mode of mothering in a particular way is, like the whole idea of maternal deprivation, intrinsic to an intellectual climate that no longer sees that human beings cannot be considered apart from their sociocultural context. A mother who is multiple sclerotic does not need pity; she needs a practical, basic regime of child care which, if consistently applied, replaces chaos with predictability, and frustration and ignorance with an ability to cope.

Reams have been written on the attachment a mother forms to her infant and, in recent years, these words have prompted various social policies. That the survival of a baby depends on caregiving twenty-four hours a day for months and years, and the survival of the species depends on the child's maturation to reproductive adulthood goes without saying. Psychologists, generally, accept that fondling, gazing, kissing, holding close and eye-to-eye contact are indices of maternal attachment. However, it is not obvious that these are crucial to infant and species survival. By no means are they specific to the mother-infant relationship; on the contrary, they are seen frequently as other people interact with infants.

Do these affectionate behaviors really explain what it is that allows mothers to tolerate, and usually enjoy, the enforced disruption of their previous life-style by infant caregiving, or maintaining contact in situations often associated with avoidance and disgust (such as feces and vomitus)? Moreover, these indices are hardly of equal importance in other cultures. For example, studies in Zambia reveal that eye-to-eye contact rarely occurs between mother and infant, nor is it reliably associated with other social interaction. Are Zambian mothers, as a result, less attached to their infants than English or American mothers?

The current research on mother-infant attachment is fascinating but it would be foolhardy to generalise the results beyond the laboratory. One fatal error a psychologist can make — and one he consistently does make — is to immediately turn research findings into a "curriculum" for "scientific" child care. The most we can say about these indices of maternal attachment is that they move us nearer to a definition of maternal behavior that is genuinely representative of our species, and to the discovery of those components that are critical for human survival. Beyond this we can only hazard a guess that it is probably not bodily care or satisfactions that are relevant to human bonds at this early age, but the amount of social interaction a person (mother, father, brother, sister, distant relative or friend) is prepared to enter into with an infant.

Even a severely handicapped woman can find diverse channels for social intercourse with her child. For example, she may choose to exploit the power of eye-to-eye contact to "hold," and no mother who is multiple sclerotic need feel a twinge of guilt about seeking help in this regard, or in delegating to her husband, or sister, or other guardian drawn from the community those tasks that physically she is unable to do. She may feel frustrated about her inability to undertake them herself, but provided a few elementary rules of child care are observed, her child will certainly fare no worse than his contemporaries. Indeed, he is likely to benefit considerably from the careful thought and planning that, of necessity, is given to his upbringing.

APPENDIX

An Experiential/Existential Approach to Sickness

PHYSICAL illness and disability are a part of life, yet we know very little about the psychological consequences of either. Nor, I believe, is this deplorable state of affairs likely to change unless an experiential approach to both is developed. For those working within the Anglo-American frame of psychological reference there are few guideposts along such a subjective route. Moreover, a rigorous training in behaviorist methodology militates against easy acceptance of the existential, European style. The first step to a genuine conversion is an experience — in my case a death encounter — of sufficient power to impel the search for a new *modus operandi.** J. H. van den Bergh, Milton Mayeroff, Oliver Sachs and, to a lesser extent, Ivan Illich and Peter Berger, have made relevant contributions in this area. My own large debt to them all, in particular Sachs and van den Berg, is quite clear. In my day-to-day work with the chronically ill and dying I still refer constantly to their writings, as well as works of fiction, such as *One Day in the Life of Ivan Denisovich.*

The experientialist looks at sickness in biological and/or metaphysical terms; that is, those of organisation and design. Every diagnostic syndrome has a coherent inner logic and pattern of its own; it constitutes a sort of cosmos. Being multiple sclerotic, for example, is a peculiar and characteristic mode of being in the world.

What is it like to be multiple sclerotic? What is the real nature of sclerotic existence? If we are subject to *experiences* as

---

*I have explored the problem of cognitive change in maturity in *An explication of cognitive change in maturity: a limited autobiographical study* (submitted for publication) and more extensively in Alpha and Omega (in preparation).

247

strange as our behaviors, delicate and imaginative collaboration between the sick person and the caregiver is needed to formulate the almost unformulable, to communicate the almost incommunicable.

"How are you?"; "How are things?", are simple metaphysical questions, infinitely simple in fact, yet infinitely complex. There are many legitimate answers in the form of statements, evocative gestures or words. *All* are intuitively understood, and each reflects the state of the person. They are acceptable answers to this kind of metaphysical question; conversely, a list of measurements regarding vital signs, blood chemistry, or what the doctor will, is not. In any event, the sick rarely describe their illnesses in physical terms. Instead they struggle to find those ontological or metaphysical words that correspond to their experience. And they talk of *sickness* as their own intimate, idiosyncratic experience and not disease. Words like "pressure," and "force," indicate something about the organisation of sickness; beyond this, they are clues to the nature of inner space, not only in the sick, but in all of us.

The dialogue concerning how I am can only be couched in familiar, human terms and it is possible only if there is a direct confrontation, an I-Thou relation, between the sick person and the caregiver.

The "pressure on the heart from the incommunicable" quickly becomes agonising in the person whose sufferings are not only intense, but so queer as to seem incommunicable. These difficulties in communication, which have become inordinate in twentieth century medical practise, arise from the strangeness, the extraordinary quality, of the person's problems, his experience. But an equal difficulty is created by the professional who, in effect, declines to listen, who wilfully adopts an approach and a language that prohibit communication. Direct questions like "Do you have this? . . . that?" are categorical in nature and, as such, demand categorical answers.

This creates a barrier to learning anything new and to forming a picture of what it is like to be as one is. Conversely, the questions, "How are you?", and "What is it like?" can only be answered analogically; that is, by the evocation of whatever is able to make the unfamiliar familiar and bring the previously unthinkable into the thinkable. It is only possible to broach the incommunicable if the sick person and the caregiver together explore and discover a vivid, exact and figurative language. Together they must create languages to bridge the gulf separating one person from another.

There are three basic ways of knowing: empiricism, rationalism and metaphorism. Each is a valid approach to reality, but different criteria for knowing are involved. Rationalism depends primarily on logical consistency; empiricism on sensory inputs and metaphorism upon symbolic and intuitive cognitions. Understanding the psychology of sickness, pain, suffering and death rests largely on a metaphoric epistemology. Here psychology is involved *in* life, not in making abstractions *from* it. Understanding is expressed in metaphoric patterns or symbol systems, those that derived from the inner space travel of the early years of life; it is not, emphatically not, in the logical statements of science. The truth of a metaphoric statement is determined by the epistemological criteria of symbols, not signs. Signs reveal a one-to-one relationship, symbols a one-to-many relationship.

The psychology of sickness and death replaces the conventional scheme of organism-in-environment by being-in-the-world or, more properly, being-in-an-ecosystem. A concrete illustration of the difference between these is the zoo. As George Leonard has pointed out so beautifully, the latter misleads us by representing the large, striped cat pacing back and forth in its cage as a tiger. It is clearly not a tiger. It is a "tiger." It has lost its ecosystem. The basic, unacknowledged purpose of every zoo is to distort our perceptions, to show us that living things can be ripped from their ecosystems and held, still "alive" behind bars and fences and moats. But *no* living creature can exist apart from its ecosystem. In a zoo, as in any total institution, such as a hospital, prison or university, it may go on breathing and digesting. It may even be tricked into reproducing. But it continues to exist only as a symbol of our collective alienation.

Disease is a functional disorder of ecologic relationships

manifest in someone who has an organic predisposition. In the world of disease, modern man no longer communicates with the sick. On the one hand, we have delegated disease to the physician, thereby authorising a relation only through the abstract universality of disease. On the other, the sick communicate with society only through the intermediary of an equally abstract reason which is order, physical and moral constraint, the unanimous pressure of the group, and the requirements of conformity.

And yet, all disease is a socially created reality. The practice of medicine consists in imputing hypothetical diseases of unknown etiology and undiscovered pathology to the sick. *All* diseases are hypothetical, *all* are labels. Faced with a "case" of something or other, the doctor seeks "evidence" to enable him to arrive at a diagnostic decision by exercising his clinical judgment. This evidence may take various forms: symptoms which form the grounds of complaint; signs which are regarded as specific to specific disorders; tests to refute or confirm the doctor's suspicions. When the requisite testimony has been gathered the doctor can say, "This is a case of such-and-such," and "The requisite treatment is such-and-such." There is, however, no such thing, entity, as diabetes or cancer or multiple sclerosis: there are only individuals who have certain experiences and physical symptoms which are said to bear some relation to the hypothetical disease.

Nor is there any such thing as a common language. Before scientific jargon dominated language about the body, the repertoire of ordinary speech in this field was exceptionally rich. Peasant language preserved much of this treasure into our century. Proverbs and sayings kept instructions readily available. But now those stammered, imperfect words without fixed syntax have been thrust into oblivion. Today the industrial worker refers to his ache as an "it" that hurts. Increasing dependence of socially acceptable speech on the special language of a technocratic elite makes disease into an instrument of class domination: the worker, Ivan Illich correctly argues, is put in his place as a subject who does not speak the language of his master.

The existential or experiential encounter between the sick person and the caregiver has nothing to do with "causes" or theories and explanations — anything, in fact, outside or beyond the helper's observations. There is no need to exceed the evidence of our senses. All that is necessary is an approach, a language, which is adequate to the subject matter. Our concern is not symptoms, but a person and his rapidly changing relation to the world. Thus, the appropriate language is both particular and general, combining reference to the person and his nature, and to the world and its nature. The appropriate terms are those of metaphysics, or colloquial speech. These are the terms of health and sickness, the alpha and the omega of the caregiver's approach.

POSTSCRIPT

THIS book was written some twenty months after I received the diagnosis of multiple sclerosis. I was a sick woman then, rapidly moving in an inexorable progression from one dreadful episode to another. In the days following its diagnosis and that of the concomitant iatrogenic disease I was numb, bewildered, unable to grasp the significance of the fact that the god I had served so assiduously had feet of clay. Within me welled a scream of protest and that iron determination to bear witness, to testify, that helps so many survive a personal holocaust.

When this urge was satisfied I knew that the Sci-Tech myth was shattered forever. The question was how to bridge the yawning gap. I began to lean heavily on existential writers such as J. van den Berg and Oliver Sachs, internalising their thinking in a way that integrated it both emotionally and intellectually. This, of course, is reflected in the "stream of consciousness" flowing through the first part of this book. In effect, then, this is a work of assembly, relying heavily on many sources — personal contacts as well as previously published material which helped me to slowly restructure my conscious self over many months. The one that emerged had few points of contact with the one that was.

Since then, however, having crawled onto the shoulders of giants, I have moved beyond this point. April, 1977, when I appeared on a national TV program entitled *Dying*, marks the start of this new era. The producer's intent was to debate the "conspiracy of silence" in which the diagnosis of an incurable or fatal disease is so often embedded. Apart from the publicity this gave to multiple sclerosis something within the viewers must also have been touched; the public response was so great that it led to the founding of what became, eventually, Pathways Institute of Thanatology. Through this I have been able to work with many people confronted by the diagnosis of a fatal or incurable disease. My experiences have led me to three conclusions which, I think, ought to supplement the arguments in the foregoing pages.

First of all why, when the multiple sclerotic is urged to "budget for a productive future, not for a fatalistic acceptance of no future at all" (see page 11), do Pathways' caregivers deal with sufferers of this incurable disease? The reasons are threefold.

Firstly, the major psychological problem in a diagnosis of incurable or fatal disease is precisely the perception of dying and death. All the lying to and by multiple sclerotics is a measure of how hard it has become in industrial societies to come to terms with death. As it is now an absurd and meaningless event, a disease considered to be incurable with no means of medical management is seen by doctors as something to hide. The policy of equivocating about the nature of their disease with multiple sclerotics reflects more than the difficulty of diagnosis; it is also a clear indication of the doctors' own fears and of the attitude that people who might be dying are best spared the news, that the good death is a sudden one, best of all if it happens while we are unconscious or asleep, as Susan Sontag observes.

Aside from the simple fact that life itself is terminal, no matter what the immortalists might say and although we like to think of ourselves as the living when we are all equally the dying, the definition of terminality is complex. Thus Pathways, in so far as it is concerned with terminal care, has chosen to work within the context of the dying trajectories of Anselm Strauss and Barney Glaser.

The first trajectory that has been identified is *certain death at a known time*. This gives the dying person and those around him a relatively specific time frame in which to order their responses. Secondly, there is *certain death at an unknown time*. In this case the living-dying interval may stretch over several years. The third type of trajectory involves *uncertain death but a known time when the question will be resolved*. Here the dying trajectory is suspended as it were because no action can be taken while the expectation of death is in doubt. Finally, there is *uncertain death and an unknown time when the question will be resolved.* This trajectory characterises multiple sclerosis and is the most problematic, for death itself is an uncertainty, and it is also uncertain when the matter can be settled. The overall uncertainty and the absence of even the prospect of medical management seems to breed a high degree of anxiety which is exceedingly resistant to orthodox psychotherapies. Moreover I am not aware that much research is being carried out to rectify this sorry situation.

The second reason is that new breed, the thanatologists, have made at least one vital contribution to our understanding of living and dying. What they advocate — caring and participation whose essence has been so exquisitely captured by Milton Mayeroff — are not, of course, new ideas. But their application to the terminally ill is. As John Langone points out in *Vital Signs,* it is entirely possible that the recent emphasis on the simple technique of being a good listener when a dying person talks may set a mood of change "in a vaunted medical system that has too long treated the disease and not the whole person, and regarded the patient as an organism, not a human being."

I have also come, very firmly, to believe with Langone that *all* sick people should have the opportunity to serve as teacher, as the dying person has since the pioneer work of Elizabeth Kübler-Ross. The third and perhaps most important reason flows from this and is the cornerstone of Pathways' philosophy regarding the gravely ill: people are responsible for themselves in sickness as well as in health. This leads naturally to a concept of self-help.

In *The Strength in Us* Katz and Bender describe self-help groups as ". . . small group structures for mutual aid and the accomplishment of a special purpose. They are usually formed by peers who have come together for mutual assistance in satisfying a common need, overcoming a common handicap or life disrupting problem, and bringing about desired social and/or personal change."

One detailed study of such voluntary health organisations

distinguished between two types of self-help groups: Type I, which provides direct services to sufferers and their relatives through mutual assistance, encouragement, education (particularly in the development of skills) and support in all attempts at coping; Type II, which emphasizes the promotion of research, fund raising, public or professional propaganda campaigns and pressure group activities at the national political level. In practice, many self-help groups, such as Multiple Sclerosis Societies, undertake both types of activity.

Neither Type I nor Type II, however, do very much to educate the doctor. Medical training and medical knowledge generally are minimally concerned with the human aspects of incurable or fatal disease. This does not necessarily mean that doctors are uninterested in such issues, merely that doctors have no specific qualifications to enable them to be particularly sensitive to these aspects of disease. On the other hand, the thanatologist working with the dying has highlighted the central importance of these human dimensions. As an extension of this, Pathways has the special function of informing the medical profession itself of the combined experience of people suffering from diseases characterised by either certain or uncertain trajectories.

Particularly in multiple sclerosis, which remains as great a mystery now as it was when Charcot identified it over 100 years ago, doctors need to rely less on research than on what sufferers say about their experiences if they are to offer genuine care to the sick. Self-help groups in the field of incurable disease are undoubtedly one of the most significant advances in western medical care in the past decade. As the spectre of iatrogenesis looms menacingly on the health care horizon, I think that these groups have a function equal to that of the laboratory in finding solutions, or at least the means of returning sufferers to an appropriate level of health. Doctors need to recognise this function of the self-help group, to promote its development and to cooperate fully with it.

A further point I wish to make within the context of thanatology concerns the central question of meaning. "It is the individual involved in and living through the state of being multiple sclerotic who imbues it with meaning." (see page 137). This is incontrovertible and applies to all diseases. However the emphasis does shift slightly when working with others. To take account of this Pathways is evolving a systematic educational approach designed to provide the adult with a deeper understanding of dying and death. I have called this thanapy and consider it to be appropriate as well for the fatally and incurably ill. Their situation differs only quantitatively from that of a person who can anticipate death at any time with some probability and, ultimately, with certainty. The defenses that protect the conscious self from the realisation of its own mortality merely operate with greater force in incurable and fatal illness.

Thus psychotherapy or counselling with people in these categories is different from other relationships. Above all, therapeutic objectives must be expanded to enable the individual to gain some cosmic dimension for his experience. The goal of thanapy then, is to help each person — in whatever state — to find in his own terms a completeness for life, a meaning for being that is not obliterated by the prospect of nonbeing. This means that the task of the thanapist is *not to try to make sense out of the disease* or other life event — only the person himself can do that — but to find meaning in the universe. This focus removes the danger of promising the person too much, or of raising false hopes. Instead it allows the person himself to discover the values that cannot be destroyed by biological death.

What this amounts to is that the incurably ill need help in terms of living and not dying. It is certainly not true that the thanatologist's full acknowledgment of the fact of death and its place in human life represents a denial of that life. Quite the contrary. The thanatologist holds that only by recognising and accepting physical mortality can the vast and rich potential of life be realised. He is also aware that only by going as quickly as possible to the real problems of the other person's life, to those questions of his existence that he has been unable to answer satisfactorily, that he can mobilise his resources in the face of his diagnosis. The immediate goal for the sufferer is the development of his own being in his own special way, the freedom to be himself without fear. Success in this depends on arousing faith in and ultimate concern for the existential Self through the achievement of self awareness.

Initially I had hoped that by communicating my own faith in universal meaning I might convince a fellow sufferer to relinquish his ambitions, his fears and anxieties and to become preeminently concerned about his own inner development. Then, I thought, he could respond with faith in himself, begin to *live*, become a whole being. But the pragmatic and nihilistic philosophy of an age that insists that God is dead cannot be underestimated. It was at this point that I began to conceptualise multiple sclerosis not so much in terms of its trajectory but rather as a death encounter — symbolic or otherwise — which, of course, any diagnosis of incurable or fatal disease is.

Many descriptions of changes of consciousness in persons facing situations of vital emergency, such as an encounter with death, or experiencing clinical death exist in autobiographical accounts, novels and poetry, but this area has been neglected by psychologists and psychiatrists. However, a systematic study of the effects of psychedelic drugs on the emotional sufferings of dying cancer patients which began in 1965 at Maryland's Spring Grove State Hospital does record such changes, and also points to possible underlying mechanisms.

By 1974 more than one hundred terminal cancer patients were part of the program of psychedelic therapy comprising three phases: first, the preparatory period to establish a relationship of trust with the dying individual and the family; secondly, the drug session itself; and thirdly, the postsession period to facilitate the integration of the psychedelic experiences into the dying individual's life.

The most important therapeutic changes as a result of this treatment were observed in five areas: (a) emotional symptoms, such as depression, suicidal tendencies, tension, anxiety, insomnia and psychological withdrawal; (b) physical pain and distress; (c) fear of death, philosophical concept of death and attitude toward dying; (d) time orientation and basic hierarchy of values; (e) grief and mourning of surviving family members and their ability to integrate the loss.

In the *Human Encounter with Death,* Grof and Halifax note that the favourable combination of several mechanisms operative in conventional psychotherapeutic approaches can account for many instances of the alleviation of emotional symptoms in psychedelic therapy. However, they do not provide an adequate explanation for all the sudden improvements observed which "appear to be much more than momentary self-deceptions resulting from altered brain functioning." Most really dramatic results were seen in individuals who experienced an encounter with death in their sessions and who reported that it felt "extremely authentic and convincing, to the point of being indistinguishable from actual dying." However, Grof and Halifax are clear that a death encounter is not sufficient: apparently the experience that "may constitute a new and powerful means for eliciting profound therapeutic changes and for facilitating restructuring of the personality" is an ego-death and rebirth sequence, followed by a unitive experience.

In helping the multiple sclerosis sufferer now I face squarely the implications of the diagnosis but emphasize particularly the psychological as well as those other aspects which extend beyond sensory experience in all directions. It is too early to gauge the success of this approach, but one thing, at least, is clear: the chronic anxiety precipitated by an uncertain trajectory in which there is still no means of medical management is radically alleviated.

24th August 1978.

BIBLIOGRAPHY

1. Alling, C. H.: Effect of maternal EFA-supply on FA composition of brain, liver, muscle, and serum in 21-day-old rats. *J Nutr, 102*:773, 1972.
2. Audy, J. R.: In Dickey, L. D.: *Clinical Ecology.* Springfield, Thomas, 1976.
3. Babbie, E. R.: *Science and Morality in Medicine.* California, U of Cal Pr, 1970.
4. Bakan, D.: *Disease, Pain and Sacrifice.* Chicago, U of Chicago Pr, 1968.
5. Benson, H.: *The Relaxation Response.* London, Collins, 1976.
6. Bernard, C.: In Feinstein, A. *Clinical Judgment.* Baltimore, Williams & Wilkins, c. 1967.
7. Birrer, C. F.: Editorial. *Psychological Scene,* September, 1968.
8. Bolen, J.: *New Age Journal,* April, 1974.
9. *Br Med J, 1*:773, 1964.
10. *Br Med J,* Editorial, 1960.
11. Burr, H. S.: *Blueprint for Immortality: The Electric Patterns of Life.* London, Neville Spearman, 1972.
12. Burt, C.: In Panati, C.: *Supersenses.* London, Jonathan Cape, 1975.
13. Camps, F. E. and Carpenter, R. G.: *Sudden and Unexpected Deaths in Infancy (Cot Deaths).* Bristol, Wright & Sons, 1972.
14. Cannon, W. B.: *The Wisdom of the Body.* New York, Norton, 1939.
15. Clausen, J., and Møller, J.: Allergic encephalomyelitis induced by brain antigen after deficiency in PUFAs during myelination. *Acta Neurol Scand, 43*:375, 1967.
16. Clausen, J., and Møller, J.: Allergic encephalomyelitis induced by brain antigen after deficiency in PUFAs during myelination. *Int Arch Allergy Appl Immunol, 36*:224, 1969.
17. Consumer Bulletin, October, 1963. In *Cancer Control Journal, 2*:3, 1974.
18. Cook, A. W.: Electrical stimulation in multiple sclerosis. *Hospital Practice, 51,* 1976.
19. Creeley, R., In Panati, C.: *Supersenses.* London, Jonathan Cape, 1975.
20. Dean, G.: The multiple sclerosis problem. *Sc Am,* July 1970.
21. Dobbing, J.: Discussion. In *Lipids, Malnutrition and the Developing Brain.* Ciba Foundation Symposium. Amsterdam, Elsevier, 1972.
22. Dickey, L. D., (Ed.): *Clinical Ecology.* Springfield, Thomas, 1976.
23. Dodds, E. C.: Protein structure and clinical problems. *Br Med J, 2*:1237, 1950.

24. Evans-Wentz, W. Y.: *Tibetan Yoga and Secret Doctrines.* London, Oxford U Pr, 1967.
25. Feinstein, A.: *Clinical Judgment.* Baltimore, Williams & Wilkins, c 1967.
26. Field, E. J.: Effect of viruses on lymphocyte reactivity. *Br Med J, 245,* 1974.
27. Field, E. J. and Caspary, E. A.: "Spontaneous" lymphocyte reactivity in the presence of virus infection. *Lancet, 963,* 1972.
28. Fredericq, L.: In Cannon, W. B.: *The Wisdom of the Body.* New York, Norton, 1939.
29. Freud, S.: Beyond the pleasure principle. In *The Complete Psychological Works of Sigmund Freud.* London, Hogarth Press, 1953.
30. Friedson, E.: *Doctoring Together: A Study of Professional Social Control.* New York, Elsevier, 1975.
31. Frisoff, V. A.: In Panati, C.: *Supersenses.* London, Jonathan Cape, 1975.
32. Galli, C., Trzeciak, H. I. and Paoletti, R.: Effects of EFA deficiency on myelin and various subcellular structures in rat brain. *J Neurochem, 19*:1863, 1972.
33. Galli, C., White, H. B., and Paoletti, R.: Lipid alterations and their reversion in the CNS of growing rats deficient in EFAs. *Lipids, 6*:378, 1971.
34. Gilson, E.: *The Christian Philosophy of St. Augustine.* London, Gollancz, 1961.
35. Glasser, R. J.: *The Body is the Hero.* London, Collins, 1977.
36. Grainger, R. G., Kendall, B. E. and Dylie, I. G.: Lumbar myelography with metrizamide — a new non-ionic contrast medium. *Br J Radiol, 49*:996, 1976.
37. Greengross, W.: *Entitled to Love.* London, Malaby Press, 1976.
38. Herbert, B., and Cassirer, M.: Parapsychology in USSR. *J Paraphysics, 6*:5, 1972.
39. Hoagland, H.: *An Outline of Man's Knowledge of the Modern World.* New York, Doubleday, 1960.
40. Hofer, M. A., and Weiner, H.: Development and mechanisms of cardiorespiratory responses to maternal deprivation in rat pups. *Psychosom Med, 35*:350, 1973.
41. Hoffmann, B.: *Albert Einstein.* St. Albans, Paladin, 1975.
42. Huxley, J.: *Evolution, the Modern Synthesis.* (revised edition) London, Allen & Unwin, 1942.
43. Illich, I.: *Limits to Medicine.* London, Boyars, 1976.
44. Kelly, R.: Management of multiple sclerosis. *Nursing Mirror, 5*:48, 1976.
45. Kwok, R.: The Chinese restaurant syndrome. *New Engl J Med, 14*:796, 1968.
46. Lifton, R. J.: *The Life of the Self.* New York, Simon & Schuster, 1976.
47. Liversedge, L. A.: Treatment and management of multiple sclerosis. *Br Med Bull, 33*:78, 1977.
48. Love, W. C., Cashell, A., Reynolds, M., and Callahan, N.: Linoleate and

fatty acid patterns of serum lipids in multiple sclerosis and other diseases. *Br Med J, 3*:18, 1974.

49. Lumsden, C. E.: The neuropathology of multiple sclerosis. In Vinken, P. J., and Bruyn, G. W.: *Handbook of Clinical Neurology.* Amsterdam, North Holland Publishing Co., 1970.

50. Mayeroff, M.: *On Caring.* New York, Barnes and Noble, 1971.

51. Majjhima, Nikaya: LXX. In Schumacher, E. F.: *A Guide for the Perplexed.* London, Jonathan Cape, 1977.

52. Meadows, D. H., Meadows, D. L., et al.: *The Limits to Growth.* New York, Universe Books, 1972.

53. Mertin, J., and Meade, C. J.: Relevance of fatty acids in multiple sclerosis. *Br Med Bull, 33*:67, 1977.

54. Mickel, H. S.: Multiple sclerosis: A new hypothesis. *Perspect Biol Med, 18*:363, 1975.

55. Millar, J. H. D., Zilkha, K. J., Langman, M. J. S., Wright, H. P., Smith, A. D., Belin, J., and Thompson, R. H. S.: Double-blind trial of linoleate supplementation of the diet in multiple sclerosis. *Br Med J, 1*:765, 1973.

56. Miller, J. J.: Discords of disease. *JIAPM, 8*, 1976.

57. Mumford, L.: *The Myth of the Machine.* London, Secker & Warburg, 1967.

58. MacDougall, R.: Circular. London, *Regenics.* n.d.

59. Mackarness, R.: *Not All in the Mind.* London, Pan Books, 1976.

60. Mackenzie, J.: In Mackarness, R.: *Not All in the Mind.* London, Pan Books, 1976.

61. National Fund for Research into Crippling Diseases: *Report of Committee on Sexual Problems of the Disabled (SPOD).* London, 1976.

62. News/Check.: *Spreading the Good Word.* 1 September, 1967.

63. Nicoll, M.: *Living Time and the Integration of Life.* London, Watkins, 1952.

64. Oates, R. K.: Infant feeding practices. *Br Med J, 2*:762, 1973.

65. Oldberg, E.: A plea for respect for the tissues of the central nervous system. *Surg Gynecol Obstet, 70*:724, 1940.

66. Panati, C.: *Supersenses.* London, Jonathan Cape, 1975.

67. Penfield, W.: *The Mystery of the Mind.* Princeton, Princeton University Press, 1975.

68. Penfield, W., and Roberts, L.: *Speech and Brain Mechanisms.* Princeton, Princeton University Press, 1959.

69. Pflüger.: In Cannon, W. B.: *The Wisdom of the Body.* New York, Norton, 1939.

70. Playfair, G.: *The Flying Cow.* London, Souvenir Press, 1975.

71. Multiple sclerosis may be lead poisoning. *Prevention,* June, 1965.

72. Randolph, T.: *Human Ecology and Susceptibility to the Chemical Environment.* Springfield, Thomas, 1962.

73. Randolph, T. G.: Stimulatory and withdrawal levels and the alternation of allergic manifestations. In Dickey, L. D.: *Clinical Ecology.* Springfield, Thomas, 1976, pp. 156-175.
74. Rejdak, Z.: Alles Lebendige leuchtet. *Westermanns Monatshefte,* June 1972.
75. Richet, C.: In Cannon, W. B.: *The Wisdom of the Body.* New York, Norton, 1939.
76. Rowe, A. H. and Rowe, A., Jr.: *Food Allergy.* Springfield, Thomas, 1972.
77. Russell, W. R.: *Multiple Sclerosis: Control of the Disease.* Oxford, Pergamon Press, 1976.
78. Sacks, O. W.: *Awakenings.* Harmondworth, Penguin Books, 1976.
79. Schumacher, E. F.: *A Guide for the Perplexed.* London, Jonathan Cape, 1977.
80. Science Editor. *The Star,* May 3, 1977.
81. Selivonchick, D. P. and Johnston, P. U.: Fat deficiency in rats during development of the CNA and susceptibility to EAE. *J Nutr, 105*:288, 1975.
82. Selye, H.: A syndrome produced by diverse nocuous agents. *Nature, 138,* 1936.
83. Selye, H.: *The Stress of Life.* New York, McGraw, 1956.
84. Selye, H.: *Stress in Health and Disease.* London, Butterworths, 1976.
85. Sergeyev, G. A.: Detection of PK by semiconductors. *J Paraphysics, 7*:2, 1973.
86. Sergeyev, G. A.: KNS phenomenon. *Symposium on Psychotronics,* Prague, September 1970.
87. Sergeyev, G. A., and Kulagin, V. U.: Psychokinetic effects of bioplasmic energy. *J Paraphysics, 6*:1, 1972.
88. Sergeyev, G. A., and Shushchkov, G. D.: The piezoelectric detector of bioplasma. *J Paraphysics, 6*:1, 1972.
89. Sexual Problems of the Disabled (SPOD): *Advisory leaflets 1-8.* London, n.d.
90. Sjöstrom, H., and Nilsson, R.: *Thalidomide and the Power of the Drug Companies.* Harmondsworth, Penguin Books, 1972.
91. Stace, W. T.: *Mysticism and Philosophy.* London, Macmillan, 1960.
92. Spain, D. M.: *The Complications of Modern Medical Practices.* New York, Grune, 1963.
93. Stern, K.: *The flight from woman.* New York, Farrar, Straus, & Giroux, Inc., 1965.
94. Stewart, G. T., and Wilson, J.: London, *The Sunday Times,* 29 May, 1977.
95. Sun, G. Y.: Effects of a FA deficiency on lipids of whole brain, microsomes and myelin in the rat. *J Lipid Res, 13*:56, 1972.
96. Suttanipata: IV, IX, 3. In Schumacher, E. F.: *A Guide for the Perplexed.* London, Jonathan Cape, 1977.
97. Suzuki, K., Kamoshita, S., Yoshikatsu, E., Tourtellotte, W. W., and

Gonatas, J. O.: Myelin in multiple sclerosis. *Arch Neurol, 28*:293, 1973.

98. Swank, R. L.: Blood plasma in multiple sclerosis. *Arch Neurol Psychiatry, 69,* 1953.

99. Swank, R. L. Multiple sclerosis: correlation of its incidence with dietary fat. *Am J Med Sci, 220*:421, 1950.

100. Swank, R. L.: Multiple sclerosis: 20 years on low fat diet. *Arch Neurol, 23*:460, 1970.

101. Thomas, L.: *The Lives of a Cell.* London, Futura Publications, 1976.

102. van den Berg, J. H.: *A Different Existence.* Pittsburgh, Duquesne U Pr, 1972.

103. Weil, A.: *The Natural Mind.* Harmondsworth, Penguin Books, 1975.

104. Weisberg, S. R.: A theoretical basis for food selection. *Perspect Biol Med, 145,* 1973.

105. West, C. E., and Redgrave, T. G.: Reservations on the use of PUFAs in human nutrition. *Search, 5*:90, 1974.

106. Wiśniewski, H. M.: Morphogenesis of the demyelinating process: demyelination as a nonspecific consequence of a cell-mediated immune reaction. In Medical Research Council: *Multiple Sclerosis Research.* Amsterdam, Elsevier, 1975, pp. 132-7.

107. Wiśniewski, H. M.: Immunopathology of demyelination in autoimmune diseases and virus infections. *Br Med Bull, 33*:54, 1977.

108. Wolfgram, F.: Chemical theories of the demyelination in multiple sclerosis. In Woldgram, F. et al.: *Multiple Sclerosis: Immunology, Virology and Ultra-structure.* New York, Acad Pr, 1972, pp. 173-181.

FURTHER READING

1. Atkinson, J.: *Multiple Sclerosis*. Bristol, Wright, 1974.
2. Birrer, C.: *The Medical Cop-Out*. Cape Town, Human & Rousseau, 1976.
3. Berger, P. L.: *Pyramids of Sacrifice*. London, Allen Lane, 1974.
4. Carlson, R. J. (Ed.): *The Frontiers of Science and Medicine*. London, Wildwood House, 1975.
5. Carlson, R. J.: *The End of Medicine*. New York, Wiley, 1975.
6. Chartered Society of Physiotherapy: *Handling the Handicapped*. London, Woodhead-Faulkner, 1975.
7. Commoner, B.: *The Closing Circle*. New York, Alfred A. Knopf, 1971.
8. Copeland, K.: *Aids for the Severely Handicapped*. London, Sector Publishing, 1974.
9. Cornwell, M.: *Early Years*. London, Disabled Living Foundation, 1975.
10. Croucher, N.: *Outdoor Pursuits for Disabled People*. London, Disabled Living Foundation, 1974.
11. Enby, G.: *Let There Be Love*. London, Elek/Pemberton, 1975.
12. Foott, S., Maot, M. L. and Mahe, J. M.: *Kitchen Sense for Disabled People of All Ages*. London, Heinemann Medical Books, 1975.
13. Foott, S.: *Handicapped at Home*. London, Design Centre, 1977.
14. Greer, R.: *The First Clinical Ecology Cookbook*. Southsea, Hants, Errand Press, 1977.
15. Hills, H. C.: *Good Food, Gluten Free*. London, Roberts Publications, 1976.
16. Jacobson, E.: *You Must Relax*. New York, McGraw, 1962.
17. Jacobson, E.: *How to Relax and Have Your Baby*. New York, McGraw, 1965.
18. Leonard, G. B.: *The Transformation*. New York, Delacorte, 1972.
19. Macartney, P.: *Clothes Sense for Handicapped Adults of All Ages*. London, Disabled Living Foundation, 1973.
20. Mandelstam, D.: *Incontinence*. London, Heinemann Health Books, 1977.
21. Mann, T.: *The Magic Mountain*. Harmondsworth, Penguin Books, 1960.
22. National Multiple Sclerosis Society, New York, in conjunction with American Red Cross: *Home Care Program*, 1976.
23. Selye, H.: *Stress without Distress*. New York, Signet, 1974.
24. Solzhenitsyn, A.: *One Day in the Life of Ivan Denisovich*. Harmondsworth, Penguin Books, 1963.
25. *Still at Home with Multiple Sclerosis*. London, The Multiple Sclerosis

Society, 1972.
26. van den Berg, J. H.: *The Psychology of the Sickbed*. New York, Humanities, 1972.

AUTHOR INDEX

A

Adolph, 73, 74
Anaximenes, 56
Audy, 103

B

Babbie, 33
Bacon, 162
Bakan, 112
Bender, 255
Benson, 146, 147
Berger, 247
Bernard, 26
Blake, 164
Brown, 186
Burr, 48-51
Burt, 57

C

Cannon, 54-55, 70, 147
Carswell, 12
Charcot, 12-13, 256
Creeley, 102
Crookes, 51
Cruveilhier, 12

D

Darwin, 121
D'Este, 12
de Milosz, 35
de Montaigne, xix
Dickey, vii, xix, 120n
Dobbing, 94
Dodds, 47

E

Einstein, 57

Embree, 178

F

Fagraeus, 106
Fessel, 152
Field, 118, 171
Firsoff, 58
Fog, 121
Fredericq, 55
Freud, 112n, 113n
Friedson, 30

G

Gilley, 154
Glasser, 132, 254
Good, 108
Grischchenko, 51
Grof, 259

H

Halifax, 259
Hare, 186
Harris, 178
Heidegger, 34
Heraclitus, 56
Hilgard, 38
Hippocrates, 56
Hoagland, 48
Hofer, 90
Hoffman, 57
Huxley, 120

I

Illich, xvi, xix, 23, 165, 247
Inyushin, 52

269

SUBJECT INDEX

273

S

Scanning speech, 13 (*see also* Multiple sclerosis, diagnosis of)
Self, 46, 55-56, 59
 auto, 151
 awareness, 58, 139, 156, 159, 164 (*see also* Spiritual awakening)
 conscious, 46, 136, 137, 157
 empirical, 46, 142-145, 151, 157 (*see also* Autonomic nervous system)
 existential, 46, 157, 159, 167 (*see also* Homeostasis)
 mechanical, 46
 social, 142, 146
Sensory loss, 229 (*see also* Multiple sclerosis, diagnosis of)
Sexual adjustment in marriage, 232-238
Side effects, 30-31 (*see also* Iatrogenesis)
Skin sensation, test of, 127
Spasticity, 228
Specific adaptation syndrome, 76, 77, 78-85, 121, 122
Spiritual awakening, 24, 38-39, 47, 58, 157-167
Stress, 62-66, 69-70, 129, 145 (*see also* General adaptation syndrome)
Stressors, 69, 146
Subacute sclerosing panencephalitis, 114 (*see also* Autoimmune disease)
Subarachnoid space, 27 (*see also* Arachnoiditis)

Sudden unexpected death, 111 (*see also* Hypersensitivity reactions)
Systemic lupus eyrthematosus, 152 (*see also* Autoimmune disease)

T

Tegretol ®, 96
Theory of evolution, 120, 162
Tic doloureaux, 87, 96
Time in relation to multiple sclerosis (rhythmic alternation of signs and symptoms), 121
Transfer factor, 115

U

University, role of, 64
Urinary retention, 197 (*see also* Bowel and bladder training)

V

Vis medicatrix naturae, 55, 129, 145 (*see also* Homeostasis)
Visualisation, 148, 151, 153-154 (*see also* Relaxation; relaxation response)

X

X rays, 127